Coagulation and Hemostasis in Liver Disease: Controversies and Advances

Guest Editors

STEPHEN H. CALDWELL, MD
ARUN J. SANYAL, MD

CLINICS IN
LIVER DISEASE

www.liver.theclinics.com

Consulting Editor
NORMAN GITLIN, MD

February 2009 • Volume 13 • Number 1

SAUNDERS an imprint of ELSEVIER, Inc.

W.B. SAUNDERS COMPANY

A Division of Elsevier Inc.

1600 John F. Kennedy Boulevard, Suite 1800 • Philadelphia, PA 19103-2899

http://www.theclinics.com

CLINICS IN LIVER DISEASE Volume 13, Number 1
February 2009 ISSN 1089-3261, ISBN-13: 978-1-4377-0495-2, ISBN-10: 1-4377-0495-6

Editor: Kerry Holland

Developmental Editor: Donald Mumford

Clinics in Liver Disease (ISSN 1089-3261) is published quarterly by Elsevier Inc., 360 Park Avenue South, New York, NY 10010-1710. Months of issue are February, May, August, and November. Business and editorial offices: 1600 John F. Kennedy Boulevard, Suite 1800, Philadelphia, PA 19103-2899. Customer service office: 6277 Sea Harbor Drive, Orlando, FL 32887-4800. Periodicals postage paid at New York, NY, and additional mailing offices. Subscription prices are $218.00 per year (U.S. individuals), $109.00 per year (U.S. student/resident), $333.00 per year (U.S. institutions), $288.00 per year (foreign individuals), $151.00 per year (foreign student/resident), $401.00 per year (foreign instituitions), $251.00 per year (Canadian individuals), $151.00 per year (Canadian student/resident), and $401.00 per year (Canadian institutions). Foreign air speed delivery is included in all *Clinics* subscription prices. All prices are subject to change without notice. **POSTMASTER:** Send address changes to *Clinics in Liver Disease*, Elsevier Journals Customer Service, 11830 Westline Industrial Drive, St. Louis, MO 63146. **Customer Service (orders, claims, online, change of address):** Elsevier Periodicals Customer Service, 11830 Westline Industrial Drive, St. Louis, MO 63146. Tel: 1-800-654-2452 (U.S. and Canada); 314-453-7041 (outside U.S. and Canada). Fax: 314-453-5170. E-mail: journalscustomerservice-usa@elsevier.com (for print support); journalsonlinesupport-usa@elsevier.com (for online support).

Reprints. For copies of 100 or more of articles in this publication, please contact the Commercial Reprints Department, Elsevier Inc., 360 Park Avenue South, New York, NY 10010-1710. Tel.: 212-633-3812; Fax: 212-462-1935; E-mail: reprints@elsevier.com.

Clinics in Liver Disease is covered in *MEDLINE/PubMed (Index Medicus)*.

Printed and bound in the United Kingdom
Transferred to Digital Print 2011

Contributors

GUEST EDITORS

STEPHEN H. CALDWELL, MD
Professor; Director of Hepatology, Digestive Health Center of Excellence, University of Virginia Medical Center, Charlottesville, Virginia

ARUN J. SANYAL, MD
Professor and Chief, Division of GI/Hepatology and Nutrition, Department of Internal Medicine, Virginia Commonwealth University School of Medicine, Richmond, Virginia

AUTHORS

S. AGARWAL, MB, MS, FRCA
Department of Anesthesia, Royal Free Hospital, London, United Kingdom

EDRIS M. ALKOZAI, BSc
Department of Surgery, Section of Hepatobiliary Surgery and Liver Transplantation, University Medical Center Groningen, University of Groningen, Groningen, The Netherlands

QUENTIN M. ANSTEE, BSc, MBBS, PhD, MRCP
Clinical Lecturer in Medicine and Hepatology, Department of Academic Medicine, St Mary's Hospital Campus, Imperial College London, London, United Kingdom

CURTIS K. ARGO, MD, MS
Assistant Professor, University of Virginia, Department of Medicine, Division of Gastroenterology and Hepatology, Charlottesville, Virginia

RUSS ARJAL, MD
Division of Gastroenterology/Hepatology, University of Colorado Health Sciences Center, Aurora, Colorado

RASHEED A. BALOGUN, MD
Associate Professor, University of Virginia, Department of Medicine, Division of Nephrology, Charlottesville, Virginia

CARL L. BERG, MD
Professor, Division of Gastroenterology and Hepatology, University of Virginia, Charlottesville, Virginia

PAULO LISBOA BITTENCOURT, MD, PhD
Unit of Gastroenterology and Hepatology, Portuguese Hospital, Salvador, Bahia, Brazil

A.K. BURROUGHS, MBChB Hons, FRCP
Professor, The Royal Free Sheila Sherlock Liver Centre and Department of Surgery, Royal Free Hospital, London, United Kingdom

STEPHEN H. CALDWELL, MD
Professor; Director of Hepatology, Digestive Health Center of Excellence, University of Virginia Medical Center, Charlottesville, Virginia

ANDREA CELESTINI, MD
Institute of Clinical Medicine I, University of Rome, "La Sapienza," Policlinico Umberto I, Rome, Italy

E. CHOLONGITAS, MD
The Royal Free Sheila Sherlock Liver Centre and Department of Surgery, Royal Free Hospital, London, United Kingdom

CLÁUDIA ALVES COUTO, MD, PhD
Alfa Gastroenterology Institute, Federal University of Minas Gerais, Belo Horizonte, Minas Gerais, Brazil

DOMENICO FERRO, MD
Department of Experimental Medicine, Institute of Clinical Medicine I, University of Rome, "La Sapienza," Policlinico Umberto I, Rome, Italy

C. FERRONATO, MD
Division of Gastroenterology, Department of Surgical and Gastroenterological Sciences, University Hospital of Padua, Padova, Italy

DON A. GABRIEL, MD, PhD
Professor of Medicine, Division of Hematology/Oncology, University of North Carolina School of Medicine, Chapel Hill, North Carolina

ROBERT GOLDIN, MD, FRCPath
Reader in Liver Pathology, Department of Histopathology, St Mary's Hospital Campus, Imperial College London, London, United Kingdom

MAUREANE HOFFMAN, MD, PhD
Carolina Cardiovascular Biology Center, Department of Medicine, University of North Carolina, Chapel Hill; Pathology and Laboratory Medicine Service, Durham Veterans Affairs Medical Center; Department of Pathology, Duke University Medical Center, Durham, North Carolina

GREG G.C. HUGENHOLTZ, BSc
Surgical Research Laboratory, Department of Surgery, University Medical Center Groningen, University of Groningen, Groningen, The Netherlands

PATRICK S. KAMATH, MD
Professor of Medicine, Miles and Shirley Fiterman Center for Digestive Diseases, Mayo Clinic, College of Medicine, Rochester, Minnesota

W. RAY KIM, MD
Associate Professor, Miles and Shirley Fiterman Center for Digestive Diseases, Mayo Clinic, College of Medicine, Rochester, Minnesota

FRANK W.G. LEEBEEK, MD, PhD
Department of Hematology, Erasmus University Medical Center, Rotterdam; Clinical Fellow, The Netherlands Organisation for Scientific Research (NWO), Den Haag, The Netherlands

TON LISMAN, PhD
Surgical Research Laboratory, Department of Surgery, University Medical Center Groningen, University of Groningen, Groningen, The Netherlands

S. MALLETT, MB, MS, FRCA
Department of Anesthesia, Royal Free Hospital, London, United Kingdom

DOUGALD M. MONROE, PhD
Carolina Cardiovascular Biology Center, Department of Medicine, University of North Carolina, Chapel Hill, North Carolina

SANTIAGO J. MUNOZ, MD, FACP, FACG
Professor of Medicine, University of Pennsylvania, School of Medicine; Director, Liver Service, PENN Presbyterian Medical Center, Philadelphia, Pennsylvania

PATRICK G. NORTHUP, MD, MHS
Assistant Professor, Division of Gastroenterology and Hepatology, University of Virginia Health System, Charlottesville, Virginia

ROBERT J. PORTE, MD, PhD
Professor of Surgery, Department of Surgery, Section of Hepatobiliary Surgery and Liver Transplantation, University Medical Center Groningen, University of Groningen, Groningen, The Netherlands

DANIEL DIAS RIBEIRO, MD, PhD
Alfa Gastroenterology Institute, Department of Hematology, Federal University of Minas Gerais, Belo Horizonte, Minas Gerais, Brazil

ANNE RIDDELL, PhD
Department of Haemophilia and Haemostasis, Royal Free Hospital, London, United Kingdom

ARUN J. SANYAL, MD
Professor and Chief, Division of GI/Hepatology and Nutrition, Department of Internal Medicine, Virginia Commonwealth University School of Medicine, Richmond, Virginia

M. SENZOLO, MD, PhD
Division of Gastroenterology, Department of Surgical and Gastroenterological Sciences, University Hospital of Padua, Padova, Italy

NEERAL L. SHAH, MD
Clinical Instructor, Department of Gastroenterology, University of Virginia, Charlottesville, Virginia

JASPER H. SMALBERG, MSc
Department of Hematology, Erasmus University Medical Center, Rotterdam, The Netherlands

R. TODD STRAVITZ, MD, FACP, FACG
Associate Professor of Medicine, Section of Hepatology, Hume-Lee Transplant Center, Virginia Commonwealth University, Richmond, Virginia

U. THALHEIMER, MD, PhD
The Royal Free Sheila Sherlock Liver Centre and Department of Surgery, Royal Free Hospital, London, United Kingdom

MARK R. THURSZ, MBBS, MD, FRCP
Professor of Hepatology, Department of Academic Medicine, St Mary's Hospital Campus, Imperial College London, London, United Kingdom

ARMANDO TRIPODI, PhD
Professor of Laboratory Medicine, Angelo Bianchi Bonomi Hemophilia and Thrombosis Center, Department of Internal Medicine, University Medical School and IRCCS Maggiore Hospital, Mangiagalli and Regina Elena Foundation, Milano, Italy

JAMES F. TROTTER, MD
Division of Gastroenterology/Hepatology, University of Colorado Health Sciences Center, Aurora, Colorado

FRANCESCO VIOLI, MD
Institute of Clinical Medicine I, University of Rome, "La Sapienza," Policlinico Umberto I, Rome, Italy

MARK WRIGHT, BSc, MBBS, PhD, MRCP
Consultant Hepatologist, Department of Hepatology, Southampton General Hospital, Southampton, United Kingdom

Contents

In this article, the authors discuss three pathophysiologic mechanisms that influence the coagulation system in patients who have liver disease. First, bacterial infections may play an important role in the cause of variceal bleeding in patients who have liver cirrhosis, affecting coagulation through multiple pathways. One of the pathways through which this occurs is dependent on endogenous heparinoids, on which the authors focus in this article. Secondly, the authors discuss renal failure, a condition that is frequently encountered in patients who have liver cirrhosis. Finally, they review dysfunction of the endothelial system. The role of markers of endothelial function in cirrhotic patients, such as von Willebrand factor and endothelin-1, is discussed.

Liver cirrhosis is characterized by impairment of primary and secondary hemostasis but it is not clear how this impairment is related to the bleeding problems seen in cirrhosis. This delicate hemostatic balance can be perturbed by numerous conditions, such as variceal bleeding, renal failure, or infection/sepsis, which may lead to worsening of coagulation status to date. The role of endogenous heparinoids (glycosaminoglycans) in the coagulopathy of patients who have cirrhosis has been demonstrated by thromboelastography with the addition of heparinase I in patients who have recent variceal bleeding and infection. The heparin-like effect has also been demonstrated to be part of the coagulopathy seen after reperfusion in patients who have cirrhosis and are undergoing liver transplant. Therapeutic implications of these findings are not clear at the moment and the use of drugs able to cleave heparinoids should be explored.

The complex coagulation defect secondary to chronic liver disease is considered responsible for the bleeding problems that often are associated with the disease. Accordingly, clinicians order laboratory tests to assess the risk of bleeding and rely on these results to make decisions about the management of the associated coagulation disturbances. Recent data, however, indicate that the abnormality of coagulation in stable cirrhosis is more a myth than a reality and may help explain why the prolonged global coagulation tests are poor predictors of bleeding in this setting. Alternative tests more closely mimicking what occurs in vivo should be developed and investigated in appropriate clinical trials to determine their value in the management of bleeding in cirrhosis.

The Model for End-stage Liver Disease (MELD) has been demonstrated to
be an excellent predictor of survival in patients who have end-stage liver
disease. It is derived from the international normalized ratio (INR) of prothrombin time, serum creatinine, and serum total bilirubin. The major use
of the MELD score is to prioritize allocation of organs for liver transplant
among patients who have chronic liver disease. Virtually every study that
has looked at the MELD score as a predictor of survival has demonstrated
that the MELD score using the INR with international sensitivity index
calibrated for patients on warfarin has a 'c' statistic of approximately
0.8, indicating excellent discrimination.

The current basis for deceased donor liver allocation is the Model for
End-stage Liver Disease (MELD) score, which is an objective means of
predicting 90-day patient survival. Although the MELD system is a vast
improvement over the prior allocation scheme, published studies have refuted the United Network for Organ Sharing statement that "the MELD and
PELD [Pediatric End-stage Liver Disease] formulas are simple, objective
and verifiable and yield consistent results whenever the score is calculated." In particular, wide inter-laboratory variation exists in the most
heavily weighted MELD determinant, the international normalized ratio
(INR). Whether this variation impacts the equitable distribution of deceased donor livers is unclear. However, the current technique for measuring the INR has the potential to detract from the expressed purpose of
MELD-based allocation, which is to prioritize liver transplant candidates
across the country with parity, using an objective scoring system.

Plasma-based products are commonly used in patients who have chronic
liver disease to treat perceived coagulopathy despite unproven efficacy
and potentially severe risks, such as transfusion-related acute lung injury,
which carries a high mortality rate. Moreover, volume expansion may
acutely worsen portal hypertension and increase bleeding from the collateral portal vascular bed. Although factor replacement therapy may be warranted in selected situations, its use should be restricted because of the
limitations of target tests, such as international normalized ratio, which
poorly reflects presence of bleeding diatheses in patients who have cirrhosis. Renal replacement therapies are frequent adjuncts in patients who
have cirrhosis and are acutely decompensated, and may correct

uremia-related bleeding diathesis and assist in controlling vascular volume, although they are generally limited to use as a bridge to liver transplantation. Novel extracorporeal therapies are emerging and may also have significant interaction with the hemostatic system. Volume contraction and blood conservation therapies are relatively new and promising approaches to reduce use of blood products in liver transplantation.

Patients who have liver disease experience an increased risk for bleeding and resulting complications. Diseases affecting the liver can cause a deficiency of pro-coagulant factors or induce a state of increased clot breakdown. Although traditional tests of coagulation, such as prothrombin time or international normalized ratio (INR), may not accurately measure bleeding risk, many studies have assessed measures used to correct an increased INR and minimize adverse outcomes. This article discusses the use of activated factor VIIa and anti-fibrinolytic agents to treat coagulopathy in the setting of liver disease and the potential advantages and disadvantages of these alternatives, and the limitations of the current literature. This article also compares the limitations, risks, and potential benefits of prophylactic therapy to prevent bleeding before invasive procedures with rescue therapy for spontaneous and postprocedure bleeding, and describes the relative advantages and disadvantages of these two approaches.

Coagulopathy is an essential component of the acute liver failure (ALF) syndrome and reflects the central role of liver function in hemostasis. ALF is a syndrome characterized by the development of hepatic encephalopathy and coagulopathy within 24 weeks of the onset of acute liver disease. Coagulopathy in this setting is a useful prognostic tool in ALF and a dynamic indicator of the hepatic function. If severe, it can be associated with bleeding and is commonly a major obstacle to the performance of invasive procedures in patients with ALF. This review focuses on the epidemiology, pathophysiology, presentation, evaluation, and management of coagulopathy in ALF.

The coagulopathy of liver disease is complex and often unpredictable. Despite clear evidence of an increased tendency for bleeding in patients who have cirrhosis, many circumstances also promote local and systemic hypercoagulable states. The consequences of hypercoagulability include the obvious morbidity and mortality of portal vein thrombosis, deep vein thrombosis, and pulmonary embolism, but possibly also include other end-organ syndromes, such as portopulmonary hypertension, hepatorenal syndrome, and spontaneous bacterial peritonitis. A more subtle contribution also could be responsible for progression of early fibrosis to decompensated cirrhosis. Future research is needed to elucidate specific mechanistic pathways that might lead to local hypercoagulation and the clinical interventions that might prevent morbidity and mortality related to hypercoagulation in patients who have cirrhosis.

Observations that hepatic inflammation and cirrhosis are associated with the presence of thrombi within the hepatic microvasculature and fibrin-fibrinogen deposition have led to epidemiologic studies showing that carriage of the factor V Leiden mutation, protein C deficiency, and increased expression of factor VIII are associated with rapid progression to cirrhosis in a chronic hepatitis C virus. Additional data suggest that this process may extend more broadly to progression in many forms of chronic liver disease. This article discusses the evidence for a role for coagulation cascade activity in hepatic fibrogenesis and explores the proposed pathogenic mechanisms including the downstream events of thrombin activation. Interference with either the generation of thrombin or its downstream activity may reduce hepatic fibrosis. Also examined are the implications for future therapeutic intervention.

Venous thrombosis results from the convergence of vessel wall injury and/ or venous stasis, known as local triggering factors, and the occurrence of acquired and/or inherited thrombophilia, also known as systemic pro-thrombotic risk factors. Portal vein thrombosis (PVT) and Budd–Chiari syndrome (BCS) are caused by thrombosis and/or obstruction of the extrahepatic portal veins and the hepatic venous outflow tract, respectively. Several divergent prothrombotic disorders may underlie these distinct forms of large vessel thrombosis. While cirrhotic PVT is relatively common, especially in advanced liver disease, noncirrhotic and nontumoral PVT is rare and BCS is of intermediate incidence. In this article, we review pathogenic mechanisms and current concepts of patient management.

Intraoperative blood loss and transfusion of blood products are negatively associated with postoperative outcome after liver surgery. Blood loss can be minimized by surgical methods, including vascular clamping techniques, the use of dissection devices, and the use of topical hemostatic agents. Preoperative correction of coagulation tests with blood products has not been shown to reduce intraoperative bleeding and it may, in fact, enhance the bleeding risk. Maintaining a low central venous pressure has been shown to be effective in reducing blood loss during partial liver resections, and volume contraction rather than prophylactic transfusion blood products seems justified in patients undergoing major liver surgery. Although antifibrinolytic drugs have proved to be effective in reducing blood loss during liver transplantation, systemic hemostatic drugs are of limited value in reducing blood loss in patients undergoing partial liver resections.

THE CLINICS ARE NOW AVAILABLE ONLINE!

Access your subscription at:
www.theclinics.com

Preface

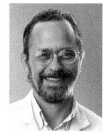 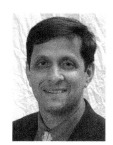

Stephen H. Caldwell, MD   Arun J. Sanyal, MD
Guest Editors

Few fields of medicine have changed as rapidly as that of hepatology in the past fifteen to twenty years. However, the management of coagulation disorders, an inherent aspect of all types of progressive liver failure, seemed to lag behind other areas for a long time and has remained mired in old dogma and unproven practice guidelines often guided more by legal concerns than by scientific evidence or rational reason. This situation has now changed dramatically over the past several years, with a number of welcome advances ushered in by landmark papers from Tripodi and colleagues, the development of new therapeutics and with it the improved understanding of normal hemostasis. Additional refinements in diagnostic tests have been greatly advanced by the pioneering work of Burroughs and colleagues. These advances have led to the appreciation of the multifaceted aspects of coagulation disorders in liver disease from *hypo*-coagulable to *hyper*-coagulable states and the limitations of conventional tests, such as the INR, to shed light on relative bleeding risk or on underlying pathophysiology in a given patient.

In this issue of *Clinics in Liver Disease*, we are very happy to present a collection of original articles from leaders in the field, and from multiple disciplines, from around the world. Each article discusses the state of the art along with its limitations. Our aim is to shed light on recent advances and to explore areas of controversy and, thus, the need for combined clinical and laboratory investigation. We hope this issue will stimulate further research on this important issue in liver diseases.

Stephen H. Caldwell, MD
GI/Hepatology Division
Digestive Health Center of Excellence
University of Virginia Medical Center
Box 800708, Charlottesville, VA 22908-0708

Arun J. Sanyal, MD
Division of GI/Hepatology and Nutrition
Department of Internal Medicine
VCU School of Medicine
MCV Box 980341, Richmond VA 23298-0341

E-mail addresses:
shc5c@virginia.edu (S.H. Caldwell)
asanyal@mcvh-vcu.edu (A.J. Sanyal)

Clin Liver Dis 13 (2009) xv
doi:10.1016/j.cld.2008.11.001
1089-3261/08/$ – see front matter © 2009 Elsevier Inc. All rights reserved.

liver.theclinics.com

The Coagulation Cascade in Cirrhosis

Dougald M. Monroe, PhD[a], Maureane Hoffman, MD, PhD[a,b,c,*]

KEYWORDS

- Hemostasis • Hemorrhage • Thrombin • Platelets
- Coagulation factors

In the 1960s, two groups proposed a "waterfall" or "cascade" model of coagulation composed of a sequential series of steps in which activation of one clotting factor led to the activation of another, finally leading to a burst of thrombin generation.[1,2] Each clotting factor was thought to exist as a precursor that could be converted proteolytically into an active enzyme.[3] The original models were modified to eventually become the familiar Y-shaped scheme that we call the "coagulation cascade" today (**Fig. 1**). The two arms of the "Y" are the "intrinsic" and "extrinsic" pathways initiated by factor XII (FXII) and FVIIa/tissue factor (TF), respectively. The pathways converge on a "common" pathway at the level of the FXa/FVa (prothrombinase) complex.

This "cascade" was not proposed as a literal model of hemostasis in vivo, but rather as a scheme of how the many identified coagulation factors interact biochemically. However, the lack of any other clear and predictive model of physiologic hemostasis has meant that most physicians view the "cascade" as a model of physiology by default. This view has been reinforced by the fact that screening coagulation tests (prothrombin time [PT] and activated partial thromboplastin time [aPTT]) are often used as though they were predictive of clinical bleeding.

Many people recognized that the "cascade" model had serious failings as a model of physiologic coagulation, and that the intrinsic and extrinsic systems could not operate as independent and redundant pathways as implied by this model. It was also recognized from the earliest studies of coagulation that cells are important participants in the process[4,5] and that normal hemostasis is not possible in the absence of cell-associated tissue factor (TF) and platelets. It is therefore logical that substituting the role of cells in in vitro coagulation tests with phospholipid vesicles[6] in the PT and PTT assays overlooks their active roles in hemostasis in vivo. Therefore, we proposed

[a] Carolina Cardiovascular Biology Center, Department of Medicine, University of North Carolina, Chapel Hill, NC, USA
[b] Pathology and Laboratory Medicine Service, Durham Veterans Affairs Medical Center, 508 Fulton Street, Durham, NC 27705, USA
[c] Department of Pathology, Duke University Medical Center, Durham, NC, USA
* Corresponding author. Pathology and Laboratory Medicine Service (113), Durham Veterans Affairs Medical Center, 508 Fulton Street, Durham, NC.
E-mail address: maureane@med.unc.edu (M. Hoffman).

Clin Liver Dis 13 (2009) 1–9
doi:10.1016/j.cld.2008.09.014
1089-3261/08/$ – see front matter. Published by Elsevier Inc.

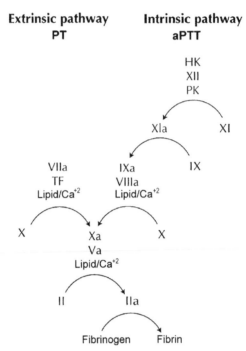

Extrinsic pathway
PT

Intrinsic pathway
aPTT

HK
XII
PK

XIa   XI

VIIa   IXa   IX
TF   VIIIa
Lipid/Ca^{+2} Lipid/Ca^{+2}

X   Xa   X
          Va
      Lipid/Ca^{+2}

II   IIa

Fibrinogen   Fibrin

Fig. 1. The coagulation cascade. This model accurately represents the reactions as they occur in the common clinical coagulation tests, the prothrombin time (PT), and activated partial thromboplastin time (aPTT).

a cell-based model of coagulation[7] in which hemostasis occurs in a step-wise process on cell surfaces, as described below.

STEP 1: INITIATION OF COAGULATION ON TISSUE FACTOR–BEARING CELLS

The coagulation process is initiated when TF-bearing cells are exposed to blood at a site of injury. TF is a transmembrane protein that acts as a receptor and cofactor for FVII. It is normally expressed only on cells outside the vasculature. TF is particularly expressed by the adventitial cells around vessels, where it forms a "hemostatic enve- lope" to stop bleeding in the event of vascular injury.[8] Once bound to TF, zymogen FVII is rapidly activated to FVIIa.[9] The FVIIa/TF complex catalyzes activation of both FX and FIX.[10] The FXa formed on the TF-bearing cell interacts with its cofactor FVa to gener- ate a small amount of thrombin on the TF cells.[11]

Most of the coagulation factors can leave the vasculature, percolate through the extravascular space, and collect in the lymph.[12] We have recently provided histologic data supporting the view that most TF is bound to FVIIa even in the absence of an in- jury.[13] Therefore, it is likely that low levels of FIXa, FXa, and thrombin are produced on TF-bearing cells at all times.[14] However, these activated factors are separated from other key components of the coagulation system by an intact vessel wall. Platelets and FVIII bound to von Willebrand factor (vWF) are so large that they only enter the extravascular compartment when an injury disrupts the vessel wall. When a vessel is disrupted, platelets escape from the vessel, bind to collagen and other extracellular matrix components at the site of injury, and are partially activated. This process forms a platelet plug that provides primary hemostasis. At that point, the small amounts of thrombin produced on TF-bearing cells can interact with platelets and FVIII/vWF to initiate the hemostatic process that ultimately enmeshes the initial platelet plug in a stable fibrin clot (secondary hemostasis).

STEP 2: AMPLIFICATION OF THE PROCOAGULANT SIGNAL BY THROMBIN GENERATED ON THE TISSUE FACTOR–BEARING CELL

During the **Amplification Step,** the small amounts of thrombin formed on TF-bearing cells promote maximal platelet activation[15] and also activate additional coagulation cofactors on the platelet surface. Although this small amount of thrombin may not be sufficient to clot fibrinogen, it is sufficient to "prime" the clotting system for a subsequent burst of platelet surface thrombin generation by activating FV, FVIII, and FXI on the platelet surface.[16–18] Thrombin activation of FXI on platelet surfaces explains why FXII is not needed for normal hemostasis. FIXa activated both on the TF-bearing cell and by platelet surface FXIa binds to FVIIIa on the platelet surface to assemble FIXa/FVIIIa ("tenase") complexes.

STEP 3: PROPAGATION OF THROMBIN GENERATION ON THE PLATELET SURFACE

The burst of thrombin generation needed for effective hemostasis is produced on platelet surfaces during the **Propagation Phase** of coagulation. Once the platelet "tenase" complex is assembled, FX from the plasma begins to be activated to FXa on the platelet surface. FXa then associates with FVa to produce a burst of thrombin generation of sufficient magnitude to stabilize the initial platelet plug in a durable meshwork of fibrin. Even though the cell-based model depicts the hemostatic process as occurring in discrete steps, these should be viewed as an overlapping continuum of events. For example, thrombin produced on the platelet surface early in the propagation phase may initially cleave substrates on the platelet surface and continue to amplify the procoagulant response, in addition to leaving the platelet and promoting fibrin assembly.

The cell-based model of coagulation shows us that the "extrinsic" and "intrinsic" pathways are not redundant. As shown in **Fig. 2**, the "extrinsic" pathway operates on the TF-bearing cell to initiate and amplify coagulation. By contrast, components of the "intrinsic" pathway operate on the activated platelet surface to produce the burst of thrombin that causes formation and stabilization of the fibrin clot. Thus, the PT assay tests the levels of procoagulants involved in the Initiation phase of coagulation, while the aPTT tests the levels of procoagulants involved in producing the platelet-surface–mediated burst of thrombin generation during the Propagation phase. Neither assay gives a complete picture of hemostatic function and neither assay includes cellular components.

THE CRITICAL ROLE OF PLASMA PROTEASE INHIBITORS

Our discussion of the cell-based model highlights another feature of hemostasis that is not obvious in the cascade model: the importance of the coagulation protease inhibitors. The "intrinsic" and "extrinsic" pathways are needed to produce activated FX on the two different cell surfaces because the presence of coagulation protease inhibitors tends to localize FXa activity to the surface on which it is formed. FXa on a surface is relatively protected from inhibition by it principal inhibitors, antithrombin (AT) and tissue factor pathway inhibitor (TFPI).[19] However, FXa in solution is rapidly inhibited, with a half-life counted in seconds to minutes.[20] On the other hand, deficiency of AT is associated with a significant thrombotic tendency. Thus, coagulation inhibitors are a critical

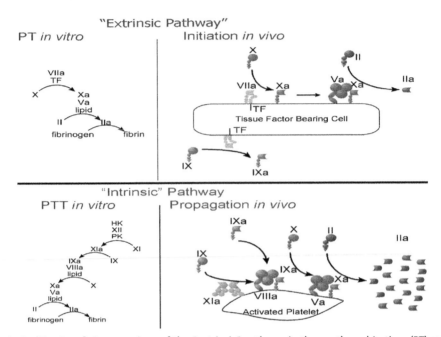

Fig. 2. (*Top Panel*) A comparison of the "extrinsic" pathway in the prothrombin time (PT) assay and on TF-bearing cells. On the left, the proteins of the extrinsic pathway of the coagulation "cascade" are shown. In the PT, relipidated TF or a tissue extract containing TF is the reagent added to initiate clotting. Deficiency of any of the subsequent proteins prolongs the PT. On the right, the Initiation Phase of coagulation in vivo is illustrated. FVIIa bound to tissue factor activates both FX and FIX on the surface of a TF-bearing cell. FXa formed by FVIIa/TF binds to FVa on that cell and converts a small amount of prothrombin to thrombin. (*Bottom Panel*) A comparison of the "intrinsic" pathway in the activated partial thromboplastin time (aPTT) and on activated platelets. On the left, the proteins of the intrinsic pathway in the coagulation "cascade" are shown, with the sequence of activation proceeding from high molecular weight kininogen (HK) and prekallekrein (PK). Coagulation in the aPTT is initiated by the addition of a charged surface, such as kaolin or diatomaceous earth, to which HK, PK, and FXII bind and become activated. Deficiency of any of the listed factors prolongs an aPTT assay. However, deficiency of HK, PK, or FXII is not associated with a bleeding tendency. On the right, the role of the proteins of the intrinsic pathway in the Propagation Phase of coagulation in vivo is illustrated. On the surface of an activated platelet, FIXa formed on the TF-bearing cell can bind to FVIIIa to form an Xase complex. Additional FIXa is formed by platelet-bound FXIa. FXa formed on the platelet surface is channeled into IIase complexes, leading to a burst of thrombin generation.

control mechanism, limiting and localizing FXa activity and thrombin generation to a site of injury. Because the coagulation cascade model was developed in an era more concerned with understanding how thrombin generation occurs than how it is controlled, this model does not assess the importance of inhibitors. As we shall see, the role of inhibitors has great relevance to certain aspects of the pathology of the coagulation system in liver disease.

THE PROTEIN C/S/THROMBOMODULIN SYSTEM PROVIDES PROTECTION FROM THROMBOSIS

Proteins C and S are vitamin K–dependent factors synthesized by hepatic parenchymal cells.[21] Protein C is the precursor of a protease,[22] while Protein S is a nonenzymatic cofactor that enhances the activity of activated Protein C (aPC). While they are often called "anticoagulant," they primarily serve the specific function of preventing normal endothelial lining cells from serving as a site for thrombin generation (**Fig. 3**).[23] This is an important function, since propagation of thrombin generation on the intact endothelium can lead to thrombosis. Thus, this is truly more of an antithrombotic than anticoagulant function.

Protein C from the plasma is localized to endothelial cell surfaces by a specific endothelial protein C receptor (EPCR).[24] Thrombomodulin (TM) is a cell surface receptor for thrombin that is also found on normal healthy endothelial cells.[25] When thrombin escapes from a site of injury onto nearby intact endothelial cells, it is bound by TM. The thrombin/TM complex can no longer carry out procoagulant functions,[26] such as clotting fibrinogen or activating platelets, but rather the complex activates protein C (aPC), which then binds to protein S. The complex cleaves and inactivates any FV that has been activated on the endothelial surface.[27] Because FVa is essential for activation of prothrombin by FXa, inactivation of FVa disables thrombin production on the endothelial surface and prevents propagation of the procoagulant reactions throughout the vascular tree. The aPC/Protein S complex can also inactivate FVIIIa,[28] but the physiologic importance of this activity is not completely clear.

WHAT HAPPENS TO THE COAGULATION SYSTEM IN LIVER DISEASE?

Because most of the pro- and anticoagulant proteins are synthesized by hepatic parenchymal cells, it is easy to understand how advanced liver disease can disrupt hemostatic function. All of the procoagulant factors except FVIII are reduced in hepatic insufficiency. By contrast, the level of FVIII/vWF is increased, often very dramatically, in cirrhosis.[29] Since all of the components in the "extrinsic" pathway are produced by hepatocytes, the degree of prolongation of the PT has been used extensively as a measure liver synthetic function.

However, not only are the procoagulant factors reduced, but also the levels of protease inhibitors and Proteins C and S are reduced in hepatic insufficiency,[30,31] a situation that is *not* reflected in the PT or aPTT. Thus, we measure only the procoagulant side of the hemostatic equation with the common clotting tests. Yet, it is the balance between pro- and anticoagulant/antithrombotic activities that ultimately determines whether bleeding, thrombosis, or appropriate hemostasis occurs.

Several groups have tried to understand and assess facets of hemostasis in liver disease. Some tests that may give a better view of the overall hemostatic balance

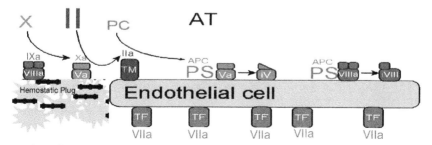

Fig. 3. Thrombin on an endothelial cell has antithrombotic function by activating protein C. The aPC/protein S complex cleaves and inactivates FVa and FVIIIa to prevent propagation of thrombin generation on intact endothelium. Thrombin that diffuses off of the surface is inactivated by the protease inhibitor antithrombin (AT).

in liver disease will be discussed in succeeding chapters. However, on a conceptual level, the hemostatic balance in liver disease can be thought of not as intrinsically pro- or anticoagulant, but rather as a state in which there is a reduced ability to maintain this balance. In other words, the coagulation system can be conceived as a buffered system in which a tendency to activation of the system is countered (buffered) by the action of plasma protease inhibitors and negative feedback loops. It is clear that the normal plasma levels of the coagulation factors are well above the level needed for adequate function. For most of the procoagulants only 20% to 50% of the normal level is actually required for hemostasis. It seems likely that this "excess" provides a margin of safety in accommodating physiologic and pathophysiologic events that consume factors or otherwise stress the system. In healthy individuals, sufficient levels of pro- and anticoagulant factors still remain after a perturbation to maintain normal hemostasis.

Similarly, when liver parenchymal damage leads to a relatively balanced reduction in both pro- and anticoagulant proteins, the net result is that there is very little change in the ability of the system to generate hemostatic levels of thrombin.[32] Thus, in the absence of a significant perturbation, patients with liver failure do not necessarily have a hemorrhagic tendency or, conversely, evidence of ongoing activation of coagulation.[33] However, when the system is stressed, for example by infection,[34] the limited "buffering capacity" makes the system fragile and prone to be tipped out of balance into either a state of hemorrhage or thrombosis/disseminated intravascular coagulation (**Fig. 4**).

Of course, the levels of coagulation proteins are not the only factors that play a role in hemostatic abnormalities that occur in liver disease. Patients with cirrhosis also suffer from defects of platelet function and number that can contribute to a bleeding tendency.[35] However, the platelet defects may also be balanced by the dramatic increase in the levels of FVIIIa/vWF, which can increase platelet adhesion and allow localization of hemostatically effective numbers of platelets.[36] Hepatic insufficiency

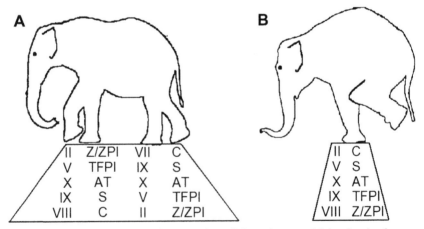

Fig. 4. Hemostatic balance. (*A*) Under normal conditions there are higher levels of pro- and anticoagulant proteins than are needed for minimal hemostatic function. This functional "excess" allows for a high degree of stability—the hemostatic balance tends to be maintained even under stress. (*B*) When the levels of the pro- and anticoagulant factors are reduced by hepatic insufficiency, there may not be a tendency to hemorrhage or thrombosis/DIC. However, the hemostatic balance is much harder to maintain in the face of stressors such as infection.

can also impair clearance of activated procoagulant and fibrinolytic enzymes, and increase the impact of any hemostatic perturbation. These phenomena will be explored further in succeeding sections.

It should be clear from the preceding discussion that the coagulation "cascade" model and the common clinical coagulation tests do not reflect the complexity of hemostasis in vivo. These "screening" coagulation tests are most sensitive to a deficiency of one or more of the soluble coagulation factors. They are very useful in defining a deficiency state in patients with a known bleeding tendency. They do not reflect the roles played by inhibitors, and do not necessarily reflect the risk of clinical bleeding. That does not mean that the PT and aPTT are useless. However, we need to understand what they can and cannot tell us and interpret them in light of the clinical setting.

SUMMARY

The coagulation "cascade" model is essential to interpreting the results of screening coagulation tests. However, it does not accurately model how hemostasis occurs in vivo. More modern models of hemostasis incorporate the active roles of cellular participants in directing and controlling the process. Different cell types express different pro- and anticoagulant properties. They localize different plasma protein components in a manner that tends to limit the activity of the coagulation reactions to cell surfaces at a site of injury. In hepatic insufficiency, a reduction in the levels of the pro- and anticoagulant proteins produced in the liver does not impair thrombin generation until levels are quite low. However, the ability of the coagulation system to tolerate or recover from an insult is markedly impaired in liver disease, allowing the system to be more easily tipped into a state favoring either hemorrhage or thrombosis.

REFERENCES

1. Macfarlane RG. An enzyme cascade in the blood clotting mechanism, and its function as a biological amplifier. Nature 1964;202:498–9.
2. Davie EW, Ratnoff OD. Waterfall sequence for intrinsic blood clotting. Science 1964;145:1310–2.
3. Eagle H, Harris TN. Studies in blood coagulation: V. The coagulation of blood by proteolytic enzymes (trypsin, papain). J Gen Physiol 1937;20:543–60.
4. Bizzozero J. Ueber einen neuen formbestandtheil des blutes und dessen rolle bei der thrombose und der butgerinnung. Virchows Arch Pathol Anat Physiol Klin Med 1882;90:261–332.
5. Hayem G. Recherches sur l'évolution des hématies dans le sang de l'homme et des vertébrés. Arch Physiol 1879;2:201–61.
6. Chargaff E, Bancroft FW, Stanley-Brown M. Studies on the chemistry of blood coagulation III. The chemical consitituents of blood platelets and their role in blood clotting, with remarks on the activation of clotting by lipids. J Biol Chem 1936;116:237–51.
7. Hoffman M, Monroe DM 3rd. A cell-based model of hemostasis. Thromb Haemost 2001;85:958–65.
8. Drake TA, Morrissey JH, Edgington TS. Selective cellular expression of tissue factor in human tissues. Implications for disorders of hemostasis and thrombosis. Am J Pathol 1989;134:1087–97.
9. Rao L, Rapaport SI. Activation of factor VII bound to tissue factor: a key early step in the tissue factor pathway of blood coagulation. Proc Natl Acad Sci U S A 1988; 85:6687–91.

10. Østerud B, Rapaport SI. Activation of factor IX by the reaction product of tissue factor and factor VII: additional pathway for initiating blood coagulation. Proc Natl Acad Sci U S A 1977;74:5260–4.

11. Tracy PB, Rohrbach MS, Mann KG. Functional prothrombinase complex assembly on isolated monocytes and lymphocytes. J Biol Chem 1983;258:7264–7.

12. Le D, Borgs P, Toneff T, et al. Hemostatic factors in rabbit limb lymph: relationship to mechanisms regulating extravascular coagulation. Am J Physiol 1998;274: H769–76.

13. Hoffman M, Colina CM, McDonald AG, et al. Tissue factor around dermal vessels has bound factor VII in the absence of injury. J Thromb Haemost 2007;5:1403–8.

14. Bauer KA, Mannucci PM, Gringeri A, et al. Factor IXa-factor VIIIa-cell surface complex does not contribute to the basal activation of the coagulation mechanism in vivo. Blood 1992;79:2039–47.

15. Hung DT, Vu TK, Wheaton VI, et al. Cloned platelet thrombin receptor is necessary for thrombin-induced platelet activation. J Clin Invest 1992;89:1350–3.

16. Hoffman M, Monroe DM, Roberts HR. Cellular interactions in hemostasis. Haemostasis 1996;26(Suppl 1):12–6.

17. Oliver J, Monroe D, Roberts H, et al. Thrombin activates factor XI on activated platelets in the absence of factor XII. Arterioscler Thromb Vasc Biol 1999;19: 170–7.

18. Baglia FA, Walsh PN. Prothrombin is a cofactor for the binding of factor XI to the platelet surface and for platelet-mediated factor XI activation by thrombin. Biochemistry 1998;37:2271–81.

19. Franssen J, Salemink I, Willems GM, et al. Prothrombinase is protected from inactivation by tissue factor pathway inhibitor: competition between prothrombin and inhibitor. Biochem J 1997;323(Pt 1):33–7.

20. Lu G, Broze GJJ, Krishnaswamy S. Formation of factors IXa and Xa by the extrinsic pathway: differential regulation by tissue factor pathway inhibitor and antithrombin III. J Biol Chem 2004;279:17241–9.

21. Fair DS, Marlar RA. Biosynthesis and secretion of factor VII, protein C, protein S, and the protein C inhibitor from a human hepatoma cell line. Blood 1986;67: 64–70.

22. Esmon CT, Stenflo J, Suttie JW. A new vitamin K-dependent protein. A phospholipid-binding zymogen of a serine esterase. J Biol Chem 1976;251:3052–6.

23. Oliver JA, Monroe DM, Church FC, et al. Activated protein C cleaves factor Va more efficiently on endothelium than on platelet surfaces. Blood 2002;100: 539–46.

24. Esmon CT. The endothelial protein C receptor. Curr Opin Hematol 2006;13:382–5.

25. Cadroy Y, Diquelou A, Dupouy D, et al. The thrombomodulin/protein C/protein S anticoagulant pathway modulates the thrombogenic properties of the normal resting and stimulated endothelium. Arterioscler Thromb Vasc Biol 1997;17: 520–7.

26. Esmon C, Esmon N, Hams K. Complex formation between thrombin and thrombomodulin inhibits both thrombin-catalyzed fibrin formation and factor V activation. J Biol Chem 1982;257:7944–7.

27. Dahlback B. Progress in the understanding of the protein C anticoagulant pathway. Int J Hematol 2004;79:109–16.

28. Fay PJ, Smudzin TM, Walker FJ. Activated protein C-catalyzed inactivation of human factor VIII and VIIIa. J Biol Chem 1991;266:20139–45.

29. Jennings I, Calne RY, Baglin TP. Predictive value of von Willebrand factor to ristocetin cofactor ratio and thrombin-antithrombin complex levels for hepatic

vessel thrombosis and graft rejection after liver transplantation. Transplantation 1994;57:1046–51.

30. De Caterina M, Tarantino G, Farina C, et al. Haemostasis unbalance in Pugh-scored liver cirrhosis: characteristic changes of plasma levels of protein C versus protein S. Haemostasis 1993;23:229–35.

31. Raya-Sanchez JM, Gonzalez-Reimers E, Rodriguez-Martin JM, et al. Coagulation inhibitors in alcoholic liver cirrhosis. Alcohol 1998;15:19–23.

32. Tripodi A, Salerno F, Chantarangkul V, et al. Evidence of normal thrombin generation in cirrhosis despite abnormal conventional coagulation tests. Hepatology 2005;41:553–8.

33. Ben-Ari Z, Osman E, Hutton RA, et al. Disseminated intravascular coagulation in liver cirrhosis: fact or fiction? Am J Gastroenterol 1999;94:2977–82.

34. Violi F, Ferro D, Basili S, et al. Association between low-grade disseminated intravascular coagulation and endotoxemia in patients with liver cirrhosis. Gastroenterology 1995;109:531–9.

35. Tripodi A, Primignani M, Chantarangkul V, et al. Thrombin generation in patients with cirrhosis: the role of platelets. Hepatology 2006;44:440–5.

36. Lisman T, Bongers TN, Adelmeijer J, et al. Elevated levels of von Willebrand factor in cirrhosis support platelet adhesion despite reduced functional capacity. Hepatology 2006;44:53–61.

The Platelet and Platelet Function Testing in Liver Disease

Greg G.C. Hugenholtz, BSc[a], Robert J. Porte, MD, PhD[b],
Ton Lisman, PhD[a],*

KEYWORDS

- Primary hemostasis • Platelets • Platelet function tests
- Bleeding • Liver disease

Blood platelets are pivotal cells in the process of hemostasis and thrombosis. Hemostasis is the physiologic process that causes bleeding to cease after injury to the vascular wall injury. "Primary hemostasis" refers to the formation of a loose platelet plug on the injured vascular endothelium. "Secondary hemostasis" refers to the series of enzymatic reactions eventually leading to the conversion of fibrinogen into fibrin, which stabilizes the platelet plug.

In chronic and acute liver failure multiple alterations in secondary hemostasis may be present. These alterations may result from a decreased synthesis of coagulation factors in the diseased liver, vitamin K deficiency, or a deficiency of vitamin K–dependent carboxylase.[1,2] Whether these alterations lead to an increased bleeding risk has been questioned in recent publications.[3–5] In patients who have liver disease, a decrease of the components of the procoagulant system often is accompanied by a simultaneous decrease of the anticoagulant system. This concomitant decrease in pro- and anticoagulant factors may explain the weak link between the severity of bleeding in clinical practice and the level of coagulation abnormalities as assessed by conventional coagulation tests that fail to test the contribution of the natural inhibitors of coagulation to clot formation.[6–10]

Recently, Tripodi and co-workers[11] used a modified in vitro thrombin-generation test to investigate thrombin generation in the presence of coagulation inhibitors. These studies demonstrated that cirrhotic patients maintain the same capacity to generate thrombin as healthy controls when thrombomodulin, the activator of the anticoagulant protein C, is added to the test mixture. These results indicate that clot formation in

[a] Surgical Research Laboratory, Department of Surgery, University Medical Center Groningen, University of Groningen, CMC V, Y2144, Hanzeplein 1, 9713 GZ, Groningen, The Netherlands
[b] Department of Surgery, Section of Hepatobiliary Surgery and Liver Transplantation, University Medical Center Groningen, University of Groningen, BA33, Hanzeplein 1, 9713 GZ, Groningen, The Netherlands
* Corresponding author.
E-mail address: j.a.lisman@chir.umcg.nl (T. Lisman).

Clin Liver Dis 13 (2009) 11–20
doi:10.1016/j.cld.2008.09.010
1089-3261/08/$ – see front matter © 2009 Elsevier Inc. All rights reserved.

liver.theclinics.com

patients who have cirrhosis is not necessarily impaired and that secondary hemostasis in patients who have liver disease in fact often seems to be rebalanced. In vivo however, thrombin generation is a function not only of pro- and anti-coagulant factors but also of platelets.[12,13] The platelet surface provides a scaffold for the assembly of coagulation factor complexes, an essential step in the thrombin generation pathway. Primary and secondary hemostasis therefore are physiologically integrated for thrombin generation and fibrin formation.

Abnormalities in platelet number and function are common in patients who have liver disease. Therefore Tripodi and colleagues[12] also investigated the effect of these abnormalities on the generation of thrombin. They found that the capacity of platelets to support thrombin generation in cirrhotic patients was indistinguishable from that in healthy subjects when platelet counts were adjusted to similar (normal) levels and thrombomodulin was added to the experiment. In most cirrhotic patients platelet numbers are decreased only moderately. Thus, thrombin generation probably is not affected to a great extent in these patients. In line with the aforementioned studies assessing secondary hemostasis, these results now challenge the assumption that in patients who have liver disease alterations in primary hemostasis are inherent to significant hemorrhagic complications.

Standard diagnostic tests of primary hemostasis such as the bleeding time traditionally have associated platelet abnormalities with an increased risk of bleeding. In fact, based on this relationship, many centers justify the use of prophylactic measures, including platelet transfusion before invasive procedures (such as liver biopsy or tooth extraction), even though no prospective studies have been conducted to confirm whether such measures are an effective way to prevent bleeding events in patients who have liver disease. Moreover, transfusion of platelets in patients who have liver disease may be associated with serious side effects, such as volume overload, exacerbation of portal hypertension, risk of infection, and risk of transfusion-related acute lung injury.[14] The recent identification of platelet transfusion as an independent risk factor for decreased 1-year survival after liver transplantation[15] emphasizes the need for a critical review of the significance of platelet abnormalities and platelet function tests in patients who liver disease.

PLATELET ADHESION AND ACTIVATION UNDER CONDITIONS OF FLOW

After damage to the vascular wall, platelets are recruited from the flowing blood and rapidly adhere to the exposed subendothelial surface. Adhesion to subendothelial adhesive proteins such as collagen requires the synergistic action of several receptors (summarized in **Fig. 1**). First, glycoprotein Ib interacts with the plasma protein von Willebrand factor (VWF), which, when bound to collagen, undergoes a conformational change revealing several platelet-binding sites. This interaction is transient, merely slowing down the velocity of platelets, but it enables platelet arrest by the action of two platelet receptors, integrin $\alpha II \beta 1$ and glycoprotein VI (GPVI), which interact directly with collagen. The interaction of adhered platelets and collagen initiates signal transduction events via glycoprotein VI, resulting in platelet activation. Activated platelets are able to interact with each other, mediated by the integrin $\alpha IIb \beta 3$, which can bridge two platelets via fibrinogen or VWF.

Platelet activation results in the release of alpha and dense granules, which contain mediators of secondary platelet activation, such as ADP, or proteins involved in coagulation. At the same time, platelets start synthesizing thromboxane A2 from arachidonic acid released from the membrane, also resulting in the secondary activation of platelets. Stabilization of the platelet plug is mediated further by the formation of

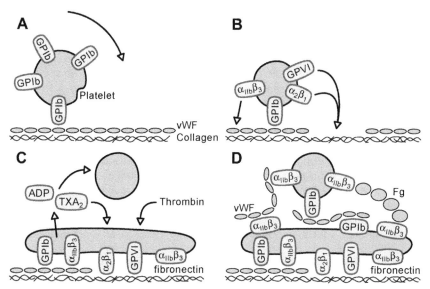

Fig. 1. Platelet plug formation after vascular wall damage under conditions of flow. (*A*) Slowing down of platelets by transient interaction of platelet glycoprotein Ib (GPIb) with von Willebrand's factor (VWF). (*B*) Stable attachment to the exposed subendothelial surface (eg, collagen) by direct interaction with collagen receptors $\alpha_{II}\beta_1$ and glycoprotein VI (GPVI), and indirectly via interaction of platelet integrin $\alpha_{IIb}\beta_3$ with collagen-bound VWF. (*C*) Platelet activation by thrombin or by platelet releasates (ADP or thromboxane A_2, TXA_2). (*D*) Platelet–platelet interaction mediated by vWF or fibrinogen (Fg) binding to $\alpha_{IIb}\beta_3$. (*From* Lisman T, Leebeek FWG. Hemostatic alterations in liver disease: a review on pathophysiology, clinical consequences, and treatment. Dig Surg 2007;24(4):251; with permission.)

fibrin through the coagulation system. As the platelet is activated, its surface alters to provide the appropriate phospholipid scaffold necessary for the assembly of key complexes of the coagulation cascade. Through a series of enzymatic reactions cell-derived tissue factor induces the formation of thrombin, which cleaves fibrinogen into fibrin monomers. These monomers cross-link into insoluble strands that stabilize the loose platelet plug.[16–19]

PLATELETS IN LIVER DISEASE

Patients who have liver disease can present with substantial alterations in the primary hemostatic system. Abnormal platelet numbers and function are common and traditionally have been thought to contribute to impaired hemostasis in both acute and chronic liver disease.[20] Thrombocytopenia is a general feature of patients who have advanced disease. It is attributable mainly to increased platelet sequestration in the spleen associated with portal hypertension. Thrombocytopenia also may be a consequence of decreased thrombopoietin synthesis by the diseased liver.[21,22] Alternatively, myelosuppression resulting from acute hepatitis C infection, folic acid deficiency, or ethanol toxicity may have a negative effect on megakaryocytopoiesis.[23–25] In addition, autoantibodies and low-grade disseminated intravascular coagulation have been related to reduced platelet survival and increased platelet consumption, respectively.[26,27] The presence of disseminated intravascular coagulation in patients who have liver disease is controversial, however.[28]

Besides the observed changes in platelet numbers, reduced adhesiveness and impaired aggregation are well described in in vitro experiments involving platelets from cirrhotic patients.[29–31] Both intrinsic and extrinsic factors have been proposed as contributing to the impairment of platelet function.

Platelet dysfunction has been associated with intrinsic factors such as acquired storage pool defects, decreased thromboxane A2 synthesis, altered transmembrane signal transduction, and quantitatively decreased glycoprotein Ib and αIIbβ3 receptors as a consequence of proteolysis by the overactive fibrinolytic system.[31–38] On the other hand, platelet function in vivo may be influenced negatively by several extrinsic factors. Abnormal high-density lipoproteins, reduced hematocrit, and increased levels of endothelium-derived nitric oxide and prostacyclin, two potent platelet inhibitors, have been suggested as influencing normal platelet function in patients who have liver disease.[39–41]

The assumption that these alterations inherently lead to an increased bleeding tendency lacks solid clinical proof, however. In addition, recent data suggest that, to some degree, elevated levels of VWF compensate for the abnormalities in platelet number and function.

BLEEDING TIME AND PLATELET AGGREGATION: DIAGNOSTIC TOOLS FOR BLEEDING RISK?

The bleeding time is the oldest test of platelet function. Basically, it is measured by inflicting a standardized cut on the volar surface of the forearm using a blood-pressure cuff on the upper arm. The reproducibility of this test, however, depends to a large extent on the skills of the technician, the skin thickness, and ambient temperature, among other factors including possible endothelial dysfunction.[42] In spite of its widespread use as a predictor of bleeding in a variety of disorders, the sensitivity and specificity of the bleeding time remain insufficiently validated in clinical practice.[43]

The bleeding time is prolonged in up to 40% of patients who have liver disease.[44] Desmopressin, an analogue of vasopressin, shortens the bleeding time in these patients, probably by enhancing endothelial-derived VWF levels.[45–47] Randomized trials, however, did not show that desmopressin had any efficacy in controlling variceal bleeding or in reducing blood loss in patients undergoing partial liver resections or liver transplantation.[48–50] This finding indicates that a correction of the bleeding time may not necessarily result in improvement of primary hemostasis. Moreover, the association between a prolonged bleeding time and the degree of liver failure as assessed by the Child-Pugh score has been shown to be independent of the risk of gastrointestinal hemorrhage.[51] These findings reflect the outcome of prospective studies indicating that the bleeding time is an unreliable predictor of bleeding in cirrhotic patients.[52,53]

In the past, laboratory testing of platelet function has proved useful for exploring fundamental processes or as a diagnostic tool for hereditary or acquired platelet defects, but standardization of testing for clinical practice has not yet been achieved.[42,54] In addition, most of the in vitro experiments assessing platelet function in cirrhotic patients were conducted under static conditions using platelet-rich plasma and leaving out essential physiologic factors for platelet activation in vivo (eg, red blood cells and shear stress) that test platelet function in a VWF-dependent manner.

The platelet function analyser-100 (PFA-100) is a rapid new in vitro test that provides a quantitative measure of primary hemostasis at high shear stress using citrated whole blood. This automated device functions with blood flowing under a constant vacuum through a capillary and a microscopic aperture in a membrane coated with collagen and agonists. As a result, the closure time of the aperture is a measurement of platelet adhesion/aggregation.[42,55] Experiments with the PFA-100 demonstrated that a prolonged closure time can be corrected by elevating the hematocrit in the blood of patients who have liver disease.[30] This finding suggests that the influence of hematocrit (and other physiologic factors) on platelet function is probably more relevant than the intrinsic platelet defects commonly found in patients who have liver disease. As yet, however, no studies have been reported that determine whether the closure time correlates with clinical outcome.

THE RELEVANCE OF THROMBOCYTOPENIA AND REDUCED PLATELET FUNCTION IN CIRRHOSIS

Thrombocytopenia is mostly mild to moderate in patients who have stable liver disease, and a mild reduction in platelet counts is in general not associated with severe bleeding. Moreover, one of the most severe forms of bleeding, variceal hemorrhage, is mainly a consequence of local vascular abnormalities as well of increased splanchnic blood pressure, and the contribution of a hemostatic impairment in this situation is debatable.[56] One therefore can argue that the clinical relevance of thrombocytopenia in most patients who have liver disease is of questionable significance. In this regard, liver transplantation is one of the most challenging situations requiring effective hemostasis. With recent advances in surgical experience, technique, and anesthesia care, however, a considerable number of patients (up to 50% in some centers) undergo the operation without the need of any blood products.[57] In line with this experience, recent laboratory data show that platelet abnormalities in patients who have cirrhosis are not apparent when platelet function is tested in models using flowing blood.[58,59]

As mentioned previously, Tripodi and co-workers[12] also showed that platelet functionality, as measured by its capacity to support thrombin generation, is not diminished in patients who have stable cirrhosis. Recently the authors' group also has revisited platelet function in patients who have liver disease, because previous studies had already shown that the abnormalities in coagulation and fibrinolysis are not as severe as thought previously.[11,60] These studies have shown that, under physiologic conditions of flow, platelets from patients who have liver cirrhosis are able to interact normally with collagen and fibrinogen as long as the platelet count and hematocrit are adjusted to the levels founds in healthy subjects (**Fig. 2A**).[58] Thus, the previously described platelet function defects do not seem to be important when tested under conditions of flow.

In addition, the authors and colleagues recently established that, compared with healthy subjects, levels of VWF are increased substantially (up to 10-fold) in plasma from patients who have chronic liver disease.[59] This increase in VWF may be the consequence of different mechanisms, such as endothelial cell activation, bacterial infection, or reduced hepatic clearance.[61–63] Surprisingly, in subsequent experiments, the authors and colleagues found a greater activation rate and thrombus formation when using platelets obtained from cirrhotic patients, who have increased levels of VWF, than when using platelets from healthy controls under normal plasmatic VWF concentrations, provided platelets in both group were adjusted to similar counts (**Fig. 2B**).[59] These findings suggest that the increased levels of circulating VWF found in patients who have liver disease may compensate to a certain extent for any defect in platelet function and for the decrease in platelet numbers.

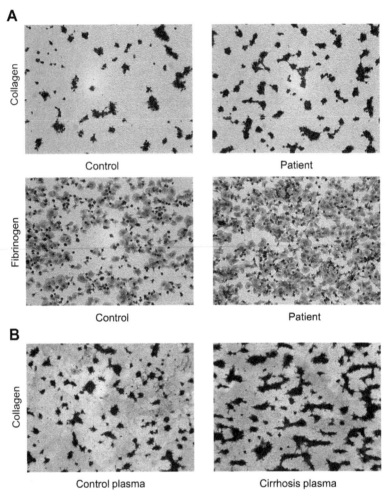

Fig. 2. (*A*) Platelet function testing under flow conditions. Representative micrographs of platelet deposits on collagen and fibrinogen formed by reconstituted patient blood (platelet count of 200 000 μL^{-1} and a hematocrit of 40%) and control blood (original magnification ×400). (*From* Lisman T, Adelmeijer J, de Groot PG, et al. No evidence for an intrinsic platelet defect in patients with liver cirrhosis—studies under flow conditions. J Thromb Haemost 2006;4(9):2071; with permission.) (*B*) Plasma from patients who have cirrhosis supports platelet adhesion better than normal plasma. Micrographs of platelet deposits on collagen formed by reconstituted blood with platelets isolated from a patient who has cirrhosis resuspended in plasma from either healthy controls or from patients with cirrhosis (original magnification ×400). (*From* Lisman T, Bongers TN, Adelmeijer J, et al. Elevated levels of von Willebrand factor in cirrhosis support platelet adhesion despite reduced functional capacity. Hepatology 2006;44:58; with permission.)

SUMMARY

Patients who have liver disease may present with alterations in the primary hemostatic system. The standard diagnostic tests, however, are of little use in the identification of patients who have an increased risk of bleeding. Increasing evidence argues against the use of the bleeding time as a diagnostic tool for predicting bleeding in patients who have liver disease. Further research is needed to determine whether newer techniques can provide a useful substitute for the bleeding time. Thrombocytopenia is moderate in most patients and generally does not result in significant bleeding events. Also the role of platelet dysfunction probably is less important than expected. Modern technology has improved the study of platelets in vitro because platelet function can be assessed under more physiologic conditions. Recent in vitro studies demonstrate that platelet dysfunction in patients who have cirrhosis is not relevant under flow conditions. The capacity of platelets to provide a surface for thrombin generation is not altered, and high plasma levels of VWF seem to compensate for any decrease in platelet function. The precondition for these experimental observations, however, is that platelet numbers and hematocrit are adjusted to normal levels.

Given the lack of data supporting prophylactic treatment with platelet concentrates before invasive procedures, and given the experience obtained during liver transplantation, in which platelet count is not routinely corrected before surgery, the routine use of prophylactic platelet transfusions when performing invasive procedures in patients who have liver disease is questionable. Exceptions include high-risk procedures in which bleeding is unlikely to be detected before irreversible damage occurs (eg, placement of an intracranial pressure monitor in a patient in acute liver failure). Prospective studies are needed to ascertain whether the group of patients who present with both substantially decreased platelet numbers and a history of severe or refractory bleeding could benefit from a therapy designed to improve the numbers of platelets (eg, thrombopoietin). In addition, the potential role of other confounding variables such as active infection, renal failure, or changes in lipid composition warrants further investigation.

REFERENCES

1. Lisman T, Leebeek FW, de Groot PG. Haemostatic abnormalities in patients with liver disease. J Hepatol 2002;37(2):280–7.
2. Blanchard RA, Furie BC, Jorgensen M, et al. Acquired vitamin K-dependent carboxylation deficiency in liver disease. N Engl J Med 1981;305(5):242–8.
3. Lisman T, Caldwell SH, Leebeek FW, et al. Is chronic liver disease associated with a bleeding diathesis? J Thromb Haemost 2006;4(9):2059–60.
4. Mannucci PM. Abnormal hemostasis tests and bleeding in chronic liver disease: are they related? No J Thromb Haemost 2006;4(4):721–3.
5. Caldwell SH, Hoffman M, Lisman T, et al. Coagulation disorders and hemostasis in liver disease: pathophysiology and critical assessment of current management. Hepatology 2006;44(4):1039–46.
6. Dillon JF, Simpson KJ, Hayes PC. Liver biopsy bleeding time: an unpredictable event. J Gastroenterol Hepatol 1994;9(3):269–71.
7. Ewe K. Bleeding after liver biopsy does not correlate with indices of peripheral coagulation. Dig Dis Sci 1981;26(5):388–93.
8. Caturelli E, Squillante MM, Andriulli A, et al. Fine-needle liver biopsy in patients with severely impaired coagulation. Liver 1993;13(5):270–3.
9. McVay PA, Toy PT. Lack of increased bleeding after liver biopsy in patients with mild hemostatic abnormalities. Am J Clin Pathol 1990;94(6):747–53.
10. Boks AL, Brommer EJ, Schalm SW, et al. Hemostasis and fibrinolysis in severe liver failure and their relation to hemorrhage. Hepatology 1986;6(1):79–86.
11. Tripodi A, Salerno F, Chantarangkul V, et al. Evidence of normal thrombin generation in cirrhosis despite abnormal conventional coagulation tests. Hepatology 2005;41(3):553–8.

12. Tripodi A, Primignani M, Chantarangkul V, et al. Thrombin generation in patients with cirrhosis: the role of platelets. Hepatology 2006;44(2):440–5.
13. Roberts HR, Hoffman M, Monroe DM. A cell-based model of thrombin generation. Semin Thromb Hemost 2006;32(Suppl 1):32–8.
14. Bux J, Sachs UJ. The pathogenesis of transfusion-related acute lung injury (TRALI). Br J Haematol 2007;136(6):788–99.
15. de Boer MT, Christensen MC, Asmussen M, et al. Impact of intraoperative transfusion of platelets and red blood cell on survival after liver transplantation. Anesth Analg 2008;106(1):32–44.
16. Ruggeri ZM, Mendolicchio GL. Adhesion mechanisms in platelet function. Circ Res 2007;100(12):1673–85.
17. Wu KK. Platelet activation mechanisms and markers in arterial thrombosis. J Intern Med 1996;239(1):17–34.
18. Lisman T, Weeterings C, de Groot PG. Platelet aggregation: involvement of thrombin and fibrin(ogen). Front Biosci 2005;10:2504–17.
19. Jackson SP. The growing complexity of platelet aggregation. Blood 2007;109(12): 5087–95.
20. Hedner U, Erhardsten E. Hemostatic disorders in liver diseases. In: Schiff ER, Sorrel MF, Maddrey WC, editors. Schiff's disease of the liver. Philadelphia: Lippincott Wiliams & Wilkins; 2003. p. 625–63.
21. Aster RH. Pooling of platelets in the spleen: role in the pathogenesis of "hypersplenic" thrombocytopenia. J Clin Invest 1966;45(5):645–57.
22. Goulis J, Chau TN, Jordan S, et al. Thrombopoietin concentrations are low in patients with cirrhosis and thrombocytopenia and are restored after orthotopic liver transplantation. Gut 1999;44(5):754–8.
23. Nagamine T, Ohtuka T, Takehara K, et al. Thrombocytopenia associated with hepatitis C viral infection. J Hepatol 1996;24(2):135–40.
24. Levine RF, Spivak JL, Meagher RC, et al. Effect of ethanol on thrombopoiesis. Br J Haematol 1986;62(2):345–54.
25. Klipstein FA, Lindenbaum J. Folate deficiency in chronic liver disease. Blood 1965;25:443–56.
26. Kajihara M, Kato S, Okazaki Y, et al. A role of autoantibody-mediated platelet destruction in thrombocytopenia in patients with cirrhosis. Hepatology 2003; 37(6):1267–76.
27. Carr JM. Disseminated intravascular coagulation in cirrhosis. Hepatology 1989; 10(1):103–10.
28. Ben-Ari Z, Osman E, Hutton RA, et al. Disseminated intravascular coagulation in liver cirrhosis: fact or fiction? Am J Gastroenterol 1999;94(10): 2977–82.
29. Ordinas A, Escolar G, Cirera I, et al. Existence of a platelet-adhesion defect in patients with cirrhosis independent of hematocrit: studies under flow conditions. Hepatology 1996;24(5):1137–42.
30. Escolar G, Cases A, Vinas M, et al. Evaluation of acquired platelet dysfunctions in uremic and cirrhotic patients using the platelet function analyzer (PFA-100): influence of hematocrit elevation. Haematologica 1999;84(7): 614–9.
31. Laffi G, Cominelli F, Ruggiero M, et al. Altered platelet function in cirrhosis of the liver: impairment of inositol lipid and arachidonic acid metabolism in response to agonists. Hepatology 1988;8(6):1620–6.
32. Laffi G, La Villa G, Pinzani M, et al. Altered renal and platelet arachidonic acid metabolism in cirrhosis. Gastroenterology 1986;90(2):274–82.

33. Laffi G, Marra F, Gresele P, et al. Evidence for a storage pool defect in platelets from cirrhotic patients with defective aggregation. Gastroenterology 1992;103(2): 641–6.

34. Laffi G, Cominelli F, La Villa G, et al. Reduced platelet thromboxane A2 production as a possible cause of defective platelet aggregation in cirrhosis. Adv Prostaglandin Thromboxane Leukot Res 1987;17A:366–9.

35. Laffi G, Marra F, Failli P, et al. Defective signal transduction in platelets from cirrhotics is associated with increased cyclic nucleotides. Gastroenterology 1993;105(1):148–56.

36. Ordinas A, Maragall S, Castillo R, et al. A glycoprotein I defect in the platelets of three patients with severe cirrhosis of the liver. Thromb Res 1978;13(2):297–302.

37. Sanchez-Roig MJ, Rivera J, Moraleda JM, et al. Quantitative defect of glycoprotein Ib in severe cirrhotic patients. Am J Hematol 1994;45(1):10–5.

38. Pasche B, Ouimet H, Francis S, et al. Structural changes in platelet glycoprotein IIb/IIIa by plasmin: determinants and functional consequences. Blood 1994; 83(2):404–14.

39. Desai K, Mistry P, Bagget C, et al. Inhibition of platelet aggregation by abnormal high density lipoprotein particles in plasma from patients with hepatic cirrhosis. Lancet 1989;1(8640):693–5.

40. Turitto VT, Baumgartner HR. Platelet interaction with subendothelium in a perfusion system: physical role of red blood cells. Microvasc Res 1975;9(3):335–44.

41. Cahill PA, Redmond EM, Sitzmann JV. Endothelial dysfunction in cirrhosis and portal hypertension. Pharmacol Ther 2001;89(3):273–93.

42. Rand ML, Leung R, Packham MA. Platelet function assays. Transfus Apher Sci 2003;28(3):307–17.

43. Rodgers RP, Levin J. A critical reappraisal of the bleeding time. Semin Thromb Hemost 1990;16(1):1–20.

44. Violi F, Leo R, Vezza E, et al. Bleeding time in patients with cirrhosis: relation with degree of liver failure and clotting abnormalities. C.A.L.C. Group. Coagulation Abnormalities in Cirrhosis Study Group. J Hepatol 1994;20(4): 531–6.

45. Burroughs AK, Matthews K, Qadiri M, et al. Desmopressin and bleeding time in patients with cirrhosis. Br Med J (Clin Res Ed) 1985;291(6506):1377–81.

46. Cattaneo M, Pareti FI, Zighetti M, et al. Platelet aggregation at high shear is impaired in patients with congenital defects of platelet secretion and is corrected by DDAVP: correlation with the bleeding time. J Lab Clin Med 1995;125(4):540–7.

47. Cattaneo M, Tenconi PM, Alberca I, et al. Subcutaneous desmopressin (DDAVP) shortens the prolonged bleeding time in patients with liver cirrhosis. Thromb Haemost 1990;64(3):358–60.

48. de Franchis R, Arcidiacono PG, Carpinelli L, et al. Randomized controlled trial of desmopressin plus terlipressin vs. terlipressin alone for the treatment of acute variceal hemorrhage in cirrhotic patients: a multicenter, double-blind study. New Italian Endoscopic Club. Hepatology 1993;18(5):1102–7.

49. Wong AY, Irwin MG, Hui TW, et al. Desmopressin does not decrease blood loss and transfusion requirements in patients undergoing hepatectomy. Can J Anaesth 2003;50(1):14–20.

50. Pivalizza EG, Warters RD, Gebhard R. Desmopressin before liver transplantation. Can J Anaesth 2003;50(7):748–9.

51. Violi F, Leo R, Basili S, et al. Association between prolonged bleeding time and gastrointestinal hemorrhage in 102 patients with liver cirrhosis: results of a retrospective study. Haematologica 1994;79(1):61–5.

52. Basili S, Ferro D, Leo R, et al. Bleeding time does not predict gastrointestinal bleeding in patients with cirrhosis. The CALC Group. Coagulation Abnormalities in Liver Cirrhosis. J Hepatol 1996;24(5):574–80.

53. Bonnard P, Vitte RL, Barbare JC, et al. Is bleeding time measurement useful for choosing the liver biopsy route? The results of a pragmatic, prospective multicentric study in 219 patients. J Clin Gastroenterol 1999;29(4):347–9.

54. Ghosh K, Nair S, Kulkarni B, et al. Platelet function tests using platelet aggregometry: need for repetition of the test for diagnosis of defective platelet function. Platelets 2003;14(6):351–4.

55. Kundu SK, Heilmann EJ, Sio R, et al. Description of an in vitro platelet function analyzer–PFA-100. Semin Thromb Hemost 1995;21(Suppl 2):106–12.

56. Sharara AI, Rockey DC. Gastroesophageal variceal hemorrhage. N Engl J Med 2001;345(9):669–81.

57. de Boer MT, Molenaar IQ, Hendriks HG, et al. Minimizing blood loss in liver transplantation: progress through research and evolution of techniques. Dig Surg 2005;22(4):265–75.

58. Lisman T, Adelmeijer J, de Groot PG, et al. No evidence for an intrinsic platelet defect in patients with liver cirrhosis—studies under flow conditions. J Thromb Haemost 2006;4(9):2070–2.

59. Lisman T, Bongers TN, Adelmeijer J, et al. Elevated levels of von Willebrand factor in cirrhosis support platelet adhesion despite reduced functional capacity. Hepatology 2006;44(1):53–61.

60. Lisman T, Leebeek FW, Mosnier LO, et al. Thrombin-activatable fibrinolysis inhibitor deficiency in cirrhosis is not associated with increased plasma fibrinolysis. Gastroenterology 2001;121(1):131–9.

61. Albornoz L, Alvarez D, Otaso JC, et al. Von Willebrand factor could be an index of endothelial dysfunction in patients with cirrhosis: relationship to degree of liver failure and nitric oxide levels. J Hepatol 1999;30(3):451–5.

62. Ferro D, Quintarelli C, Lattuada A, et al. High plasma levels of von Willebrand factor as a marker of endothelial perturbation in cirrhosis: relationship to endotoxemia. Hepatology 1996;23(6):1377–83.

63. Hollestelle MJ, Geertzen HG, Straatsburg IH, et al. Factor VIII expression in liver disease. Thromb Haemost 2004;91(2):267–75.

Hyperfibrinolysis in Liver Disease

Domenico Ferro, MD[a,b,*], Andrea Celestini, MD[b], Francesco Violi, MD[b]

KEYWORDS

- Hyperfibrinolysis • tPA • Liver disease • Variceal bleeding
- Liver transplantation • Aprotinin

The association between liver disease and accelerated fibrinolysis was described more than 80 years ago when the rapid reliquidification of incubated, clotted blood from cirrhotic patients was noted.[1] In the current literature the occurrence of hyperfibrinolysis in patients who have cirrhosis has been suggested but is still debated.[2] The reasons for this uncertainty probably lie in the lack of appropriate laboratory tests for the evaluation of hyperfibrinolysis.[3] Thus, the assay of individual components rather than evaluation of the overall fibrinolytic activity has been investigated.[3–5] Nonetheless, there is a relative consensus that hyperfibrinolysis may complicate the clinical course of patients who have cirrhosis or liver failure.[6–9] In a previous study the incidence of hyperfibrinolysis, diagnosed by abnormal euglobulin lysis time, was 36%,[10] comparable to most,[7,11] but not all, previous reports[12] in patients who underwent liver transplantation. Hyperfibrinolysis correlated positively with the severity of underlying liver disease (the Child-Pugh classification),[10,13–15] and low-grade systemic fibrinolysis was found in 30% to 46% of patients who had end-stage liver disease.[16] Therefore the debate regarding hyperfibrinolysis in liver disease focused essentially on the mechanism of hyperfibrinolysis and its role, if any, in the bleeding disorders complicating the clinical course of liver cirrhosis.

PATHOPHYSIOLOGY OF HYPERFIBRINOLYSIS IN LIVER DISEASE
Imbalance of the Fibrinolytic System

All the proteins involved in fibrinolysis, except for tissue plasminogen activator (tPA) and plasminogen activator inhibitor 1 (PAI-1), are synthesized in the liver.[17] Reduced plasma levels of plasminogen,[18] alpha2-antiplasmin,[19–21] histidine-rich-glycoprotein,[22,23] and factor XIII[24] are found in cirrhosis. There is general agreement that patients who have liver cirrhosis have increased values of tPA[13,25–27] that

[a] Department of Experimental Medicine, University of Rome, "La Sapienza", Rome, Italy
[b] Institute of Clinical Medicine I, University of Rome, "La Sapienza", Policlinico Umberto I, 00181 Rome, Italy
* Corresponding author. Institute of Clinical Medicine I, University of Rome, "La Sapienza", Policlinico Umberto I, 00181 Rome, Italy.
E-mail address: mimmo.ferro@virgilio.it (D. Ferro).

Clin Liver Dis 13 (2009) 21–31
doi:10.1016/j.cld.2008.09.008
1089-3261/08/$ – see front matter © 2009 Elsevier Inc. All rights reserved.

probably result from reduced hepatic clearance,[28,29] but the measure of plasminogen activator inhibitor type 1 (PAI-1) gives conflicting results[3,25,30,31] and seems to be influenced greatly by the characteristics of the patients screened. Thus, circulating levels of PAI-1 are elevated in patients who have chronic liver disease,[13,32] but they are depressed in severe liver failure.[13,33] It has been suggested that, in patients who have severe liver failure, hyperfibrinolysis occurs when plasminogen activation by tPA is accelerated on the fibrin surface, and decreased levels of PAI-1 and alpha2-antiplasmin fail to balance it. In contrast, there are high levels of the acute-phase reactant PAI-1, leading to a shift toward hypofibrinolysis in acute liver failure.[8]

In the last few years, another plasma protein, thrombin-activatable fibrinolysis inhibitor (TAFI), has been identified. It is synthesized by the liver and plays an important regulatory role in fibrinolysis.[34–36] Upon activation by thrombin or plasmin, it is converted to an enzyme (TAFIa) with carboxypeptidase B–like activity that inhibits fibrinolysis through the removal of C-terminal lysines from partially degraded fibrin.[37,38] Particular attention has been focused on TAFI on the assumption that its decreased levels might account for hyperfibrinolysis in cirrhosis.[39] Lisman and colleagues[40] tested this hypothesis by measuring the individual components of fibrinolysis and by using a global test to assess the overall plasmatic fibrinolytic capacity. They concluded that the deficiency of TAFI in cirrhotic patients is not associated with increased plasma fibrinolysis resulting from the concomitant reduction of profibrinolytic factors. Colucci and colleagues,[41] however, showed TAFI antigen and activity levels are reduced markedly in cirrhotic patients and concluded that in vitro plasma hyperfibrinolysis is caused largely by defective TAFIa generation resulting from low TAFI levels. These different results probably can be explained by the different designs of the global fibrinolysis assays performed in the two studies. A recent report described a new method for assessing the global fibrinolytic capacity of both the extrinsic and the intrinsic pathway and confirmed the presence of hyperfibrinolysis in chronic liver disease.[42]

At the origin of hyperfibrinolytic state in liver cirrhosis, physiologic stress, including infection, may be involved through the increased release of tPA.[43] Extravascular activation of the fibrinolytic system also has been suggested as playing a role. Ascites has fibrinolytic activity,[44] and its absorption could affect systemic fibrinolysis. Thus, because ascites fluid re-enters the systemic circulation via the thoracic duct (a natural peritoneovenous shunt with up to 20 L reabsorbed daily), this phenomenon could be a trigger for accelerated fibrinolysis.

Accelerated Intravascular Coagulation and Fibrinolysis

The significance of low-grade disseminated intravascular coagulation in liver cirrhosis is another debated issue.[33,45–49] As with hyperfibrinolysis, the variable characteristics of the patients screened may explain the divergent results. Thus, with the use of highly sensitive tests such as prothrombin fragment 1+2 (a marker of in vivo thrombin generation), D-dimer (a product of thrombin and plasmin activation), high-molecular-weight fibrin/fibrinogen complexes, or soluble fibrin, a particular profile, accelerated intravascular coagulation and fibrinolysis (AICF), was detected in about 30% of cirrhotics, depending on the degree of liver failure.[2,49,50] AICF seems to occur predominantly in patients who have moderate-to-severe liver failure but is not detected in compensated patients[51] AICF probably results from the formation of a fibrin clot that is more susceptible to plasmin degradation because of elevated levels of tPA or the presence of dysfibrinogen. A reduced release of PAI to control tPA and lack of alpha2-antiplasmin to quench plasmin activity promotes secondary hyperfibrinolysis.

An additional stress, such as infection, may influence these processes with a consequent imbalance of the clotting and fibrinolytic system.[3] In patients who have acute or chronic liver disease, an impairment of the reticuloendothelial system and/or the presence of portosystemic shunts may lead, in the absence of sepsis, to enhanced endotoxemia into the systemic circulation.[52] In decompensated liver cirrhosis, high levels of circulating endotoxin were correlated with monocyte expression of tissue factor mRNA, prothrombin factor 1+2, and D-dimer, suggesting a direct relationship between clotting activation and endotoxemia.[53,54] This hypothesis was supported by the decrease of clotting and fibrinolytic activation after the reduction of endotoxemia obtained with nonabsorbable antibiotics.[54]

HYPERFIBRINOLYSIS AND BLEEDING

Bleeding is a frequent and often severe complication of liver cirrhosis.[55] Variceal hemorrhage occurs at a yearly rate of 5% to 15%. The most important predictor of hemorrhage is the size of varices. Patients who have large varices are at the highest risk of first hemorrhage (15% per year).[56] Other predictors of hemorrhage are decompensated cirrhosis and the endoscopic presence of red wale marks.[56] Bleeding from esophageal varices is associated with a mortality of at least 20% at 6 weeks,[57–59] and late rebleeding occurs in approximately 60% of untreated patients, generally within 1 or 2 years of the index hemorrhage.[60,61] Hemodynamic alterations secondary to portal hypertension are considered the main cause of gastrointestinal bleeding in cirrhotics.[62,63] The role played by the coagulopathy of cirrhosis in gastrointestinal bleeding is still unclear.[64,65] Coagulopathy does not seem to play a major role in initiating bleeding, but a relationship between severity of bleeding and coagulation defects has been postulated.[13] Variceal bleeding is more severe, more difficult to control, and more likely to recur in patients who have advanced liver failure, which presents as defects of primary and secondary hemostasis.[66,67] Otherwise, the recent literature indicates the hemostatic changes either impair or promote hemostasis, thus suggesting a rebalanced hemostatic system in liver disease.[17]

Previous studies suggested that hyperfibrinolysis may be a good predictor of gastrointestinal bleeding.[68,69] Consistent with these preliminary reports, the authors demonstrated that fibrinogen degradation products in the serum increase the risk of bleeding in cirrhosis;[70] however, the methodologic problems related to this assay rendered these data difficult to interpret.[46] In another report, hyperfibrinolysis, as assessed by high values of D-dimer and tPA activity, was found to be a predictor of the first episode of upper gastrointestinal bleeding in cirrhotic patients who had portal hypertension.[71] Hyperfibrinolysis was associated closely with the degree of liver failure and ascites and constituted a further risk, in addition to variceal size, in predicting gastrointestinal bleeding.[71] The interference of hyperfibrinolysis with clotting activation and platelet function might account for this association. Thus, as a consequence of hyperfibrinolysis, clotting activation may be delayed because of the consumption of clotting factor and inhibition of fibrin polymerization.[72] Hyperfibrinolysis also reduces platelet adhesion and aggregation by degradation of von Willebrand's factor and fibrinogen platelet receptors (glycoprotein Ib and IIb/IIIa).[73,74] Finally, hyperfibrinolysis may provoke clot lysis by inducing platelet disaggregation and disruption of the hemostatic plug.[75]

These arguments suggest that when esophageal varices rupture, hyperfibrinolysis may delay primary hemostasis or clotting activation or induce disruption of the hemostatic plug, thereby aggravating variceal bleeding and increasing the likelihood of recurrence.[73,76]

HYPERFIBRINOLYSIS IN LIVER TRANSPLANTATION

In earlier studies, up to 75% of liver transplantations required a blood transfusion, and the mortality and morbidity at 1 year were related closely to the quantity of blood components required.[77] Although refinements in surgical techniques have reduced the need for blood transfusions, this population remains at a significant risk of bleeding problems. Since the 1960s, alterations in hemostatic system and activation of fibrinolysis pathway have been considered to be responsible for a hemorrhagic diathesis.[78] The risk of bleeding in the preanhepatic stage is related directly to the preoperative hemorrhagic risk related to the underlying liver disease. During this phase, in fact, there usually are no changes in the hemostatic profile, and there are no significant differences between liver transplantation and other abdominal interventions in cirrhotic patients.

During the second anhepatic stage, a veno-venous bypass maintains venous return, and most vessels are clamped off; so there is no hepatic function and no risk of surgical bleeding. Life-threatening blood loss may occur, however. Many studies have reported enhanced fibrinolytic activity during this period,[79] and the lack of tPA clearance and the reduction of $\alpha2$-antiplasmin may be responsible for enhanced primary fibrinolysis.[49]

Reperfusion of the liver during the postanhepatic phase is the crucial point of the intervention; although the surgical trauma is comparable to the previous stages, the amount of blood loss is completely different. Some patients may present with uncontrollable diffuse bleeding within a few minutes after reperfusion. Primary fibrinolysis seems to play a pivotal role in this phase also.[49,78] Porte and colleagues[12] demonstrated that the rise of tPA during the anhepatic phase is followed by a dramatic increase after reperfusion in almost three quarters of patients who undergo liver transplantation. Usually hyperfibrinolysis subsides within an hour, but in damaged donor liver a sustained increased fibrinolytic activity may be observed.[80] The endothelium of the donor liver is an important source of tPA; the ischemic damage to the graft during preservation may explain the dramatic increase in plasminogen activators. In the postoperative period, a reduction in platelet count is related to blood loss. Both thrombopoietin plasma levels and an increase in platelet consumption contribute to the development of thrombocytopenia. The platelet count usually normalizes after 2 weeks.[81]

The monitoring of coagulation and fibrinolysis activity is an essential element of care during liver transplantation. Among the diagnostic tests usually performed (listed in **Table 1**), thromboelastography highlights alterations at every step in the cascade from clot formation to its lysis (see also the article by A. Tripodi in this issue). Thus with thromboelastography it is possible to know if bleeding results from a failure to provide adequate surgical hemostasis, whether there are platelet dysfunction or anomalies in coagulation proteases or their inhibitors, and whether the blood loss is associated with early, excessive fibrinolysis. Finally, thromboelastography allows a rational approach to the correct used of blood components in transfusion or drug therapy.[82]

THERAPY

Antihyperfibrinolytic therapy is an important component of hemostatic therapy in hepatic diseases (see also the article by Shah and Berg in this issue). Both ε–aminocaproic acid (EACA) and tranexamic acid interfere with the plasminogen binding to the fibrin, reducing the conversion of plasminogen to plasmin; although EACA and tranexamic acid have been used widely to prevent blood loss during liver

Table 1
Diagnostic tests in hyperfibrinolysis

Laboratory Test	Methodology	Normal Range	Limitation
Clot lysis time	In vitro clot dissolution	30–60 minutes	High interindividual variability
Euglobin lysis time	In vitro clot dissolution without plasmin inhibitors	5–27 hours	High interindividual variability
D-dimer assay	Determination by latex immunoagglutination assay	0.0–0.4 μg fibrinogen equivalent/mL	Low specificity
Fibrinogen degradation products assay	Determination by latex immunoagglutination assay	< 5 μg/mL	Low specificity
tPA assay	Binding to the wells of a microtiter plate by anti-tPA monoclonal antibodies	0.2–2.0 IU/mL	Requires specific tube
Thromboelastogram clot lysis index	Thromboelastography	Amplitude at 60 minutes as a percentage of the maximal amplitude (< 40%)	Requires a thromboelastogram

transplantation, the evidence base for their efficacy is limited. Only a single randomized trial, performed 20 years ago,[11] demonstrated the efficacy of EACA in reducing blood cell transfusion; moreover studies testing the usefulness of tranexamic acid have reported divergent results; trials that used high dosage (40 mg/kg/hour), reported a significant reduction of bleeding,[83] but no efficacy was found when this drug was used at lower dosages.[84] Thromboembolic complications may occur with a high-dose regimen, and the optimal dose of tranexamic acid for orthotopic liver transplantation is still unknown.

Aprotinin is a serin-protease inhibitor that reduces fibrinolytic activity by inhibiting plasmin and kallicrein.[85] This drug has been used in liver transplantation since 1990. Because randomized trials have shown a reduction in the need for blood transfusion of about 30%,[86] aprotinin now is the most widely used antifibrinolytic drug during liver transplantation. It is usually administered as 2×10^6 units over 30 minutes followed by continuous infusion of 0.5×10^6 units/hour. Aprotinin and other antifibrinolytic agents are potentially associated with two important complications: the development of thromboembolic events and the induction of acute renal tubular necrosis. A recent meta-analysis that included almost 1500 patients, however, demonstrated that the administration of antifibrinolytic therapy during liver transplantation is not significantly associated with an increased risk of thromboembolism.[87] Similarly, a recent randomized trial that enrolled about 1000 patients demonstrated that aprotinin is associated with a major risk of developing transient renal dysfunction during the first days after orthotopic liver transplantation, but it is not associated with a long-term renal disease or increased mortality.[88]

SUMMARY

Although it has been difficult to assess its overall magnitude, and debate remains, there is a relative consensus that hyperfibrinolysis can complicate the overall clinical course of liver cirrhosis, especially in cases of moderate-to-severe liver failure. Primary imbalance of the fibrinolytic system seems to be related to higher circulating levels of tPA, but accelerated intravascular coagulation with secondary hyperfibrinolysis also has been reported overall in patients who have liver failure. Hyperfibrinolysis may delay primary hemostasis, thereby aggravating variceal bleeding and making recurrence more likely. Liver transplantation may be associated with a dramatic increase in fibrinolytic activity, especially during the reperfusion phase; thus, some patients may present with uncontrollable bleeding, requiring blood transfusion and specific antifibrinolytic therapy. At present, aprotinin, a plasmin inhibitor, is the most widely used antifibrinolytic drug, because it reduces the need for blood transfusion by about 30%; moreover, although the use antifibrinolytic drugs may be related to thromboembolic events and the occurrence of renal tubular necrosis, recent evidence has demonstrated that the use of aprotinin is not associated with these adverse events.

REFERENCES

1. Goodpasture EW. Fibrinolysis in chronic hepatic insufficiency. Bull Johns Hoppkins Hosp 1914;25:330–2.
2. Caldwell SH, Hoffman M, Lisman T, et al. Coagulation disorders and hemostasis in liver disease: pathophysiology and critical assessment of current management. Hepatology 2006;44:1039–46.

3. Tripodi A, Mannucci PM. Abnormalities of hemostasis in chronic liver disease: reappraisal of their clinical significance and need for clinical and laboratory research. J Hepatol 2007;46:727–33.

4. Brodsky I, Dennis LH. Evaluation of fibrinolysis in hepatic cirrhosis. Relation of serial thrombin time and euglobulin lysis time. Am J Clin Pathol 1966;45:61–9.

5. Glassman A, Abram M, Baxter G, et al. Euglobulin lysis times: an update. Ann Clin Lab Sci 1993;23:329–32.

6. Broohy MT, Fiore L, Deykin D. Hemostasis. In: Zakim D, Boyer TD, editors. Hepatology: a textbook of liver disease, 3rd edition. Philadelphia: Saunders 1196:691–719.

7. Steib A, Gengenwin AS, Freys G, et al. Predictive factors of hyperfibrinolytic activity during liver transplantation in cirrhotic patients. Br J Anaesth 1994;73:645–8.

8. Pernambuco JR, Langley PG, Hughes RD, et al. Activation of the fibrinolytic system in patients with fulminant liver failure. Hepatology 1993;18:1350–6.

9. Gunawan B, Runyon B. The efficacy and safety of e-aminocaproic acid treatment in patients with cirrhosis and hyperfibrinolysis. Aliment Pharmacol Ther 2006;23:115–20.

10. Hu KQ, Yu AS, Tyyagura L, et al. Hyperfibrinolytic activity in hospitalized cirrhotic patients in a referral liver unit. Am J Gastroenterol 2001;96:1581–6.

11. Kang Y, Lewis JH, Navalgund A, et al. Epsilon-aminocaproic acid for treatment of fibrinolysis during liver transplantation. Anesthesiology 1987;66:766–73.

12. Porte RJ, Bontempo FA, Knot EA, et al. Systemic effects of tissue plasminogen activator-associated fibrinolysis and its relation to thrombin generation in orthotopic liver transplantation. Transplantation 1989;47:978–84.

13. Boks AL, Brommer EJ, Schalm SW, et al. Hemostasis and fibrinolysis in severe liver failure and their relation to hemorrhage. Hepatology 1986;6:79–86.

14. Leebek FW, Kluft C, Knot EA, et al. A shift in balance between profibrinolytic and antifibrinolytic factors causes enhanced fibrinolysis in cirrhosis. Gastroenterology 1991;101:1382–90.

15. Ferro D, Quintarelli C, Saliola M, et al. Prevalence of hyperfibrinolysis in patients with liver cirrhosis. Fibrinolysis 1993;7:59–62.

16. Kujovich JL. Hemostatic defects in end stage liver disease. Crit Care Clin 2005; 21:563–87.

17. Lisman T, Leebek FWG. Hemostatic alterations in liver disease: a review on pathophysiology, clinical consequences, and treatment. Dig Surg 2007;24:250–8.

18. Stein SF, Harker LA. Kinetic and functional studies of platelets, fibrinogen and plasminogen in patients with hepatic cirrhosis. J Lab Clin Med 1982;99:217–30.

19. Aoki N, Yamamata T. The alpha-2 plasmin inhibitor levels in liver disease. Clin Chim Acta 1978;84:99–105.

20. Ea Knot, Drijfhout HR, tenCate JW, et al. Alpha 2-plamin inhibitor metabolism in patients with liver cirrhosis. J Lab Clin Med 1985;105:353–8.

21. Marongiu F, Mamusa AM, Mameli G, et al. Alpha 2 antiplasmin and disseminated intravascular coagulation in liver cirrhosis. Thromb Res 1985;37:287–94.

22. Gram J, Jespersen J, Ingeberg S, et al. Plasma histidine-rich glycoprotein and plasminogen in patients with liver disease. Thromb Res 1985;39:411–7.

23. Leebek FW, Kluft C, Knot EA, et al. Histidine-rich glycoprotein is elevated in mild liver cirrhosis and decreased in moderate and severe liver cirrhosis. J Lab Clin Med 1989;113:493–7.

24. Biland L, Duckert F, prisender S, et al. Quantitative estimation of coagulation factors in liver disease. The diagnostic and prognostic value of factor XIII, factor V and plasminogen. Thromb Haemost 1978;39:646–56.

25. Sl Hersch, Kunelis T, Francis RB. The pathogenesis of accelerated fibrinolysis in liver cirrhosis. A critical role for plasminogen activator inhibitor. Blood 1987;69: 1315–9.
26. Na Booth, Andersen JA, Bennet B. Plasminogen activators in alcoholic cirrhosis: demonstration of increased tissue-type and urokinase-type activator. J Clin Pathol 1984;37:772–7.
27. Lasierra J, Aza MJ, Vilades E, et al. Tissue plasminogen activator and plasminogen activator inhibitor in patients with liver cirrhosis. Fibrinolysis 1991; 5:117–20.
28. Rijken DC, Emeis JJ. Clearance of the heavy and light polypeptide chains of human tissue-type plasminogen activators in rats. Biochem J 1986;238:643–6.
29. Einarasson M, Smedsrod B, Pertoft H. Uptake and degradation of tissue plasminogen activator in rats liver. Thromb Haemost 1988;59:474–9.
30. TS Sinclair, Booth NA, Penman SM, et al. Protease inhibitors in liver disease. Scand J Gastroenterol 1988;23:620–4.
31. Huber K, Kirchheimer JC, Korninger C, et al. Hepatic synthesis and clearance of components of the fibrinolytic system in healthy volunteers and in patients with different stages of liver cirrhosis. Thromb Res 1991;62:491–500.
32. Tran-Thang C, Fasel-Felley J, Pralong G. Plasminogen activators and plasminogen activator inhibitors in liver deficiencies caused by chronic alcoholism or infectious hepatitis. Thromb Haemost 1989;62:651–3.
33. Violi F, Ferro D, Basili S, et al. Hyperfibrinolysis resulting from clotting activation in patients with different degrees of cirrhosis. Hepatology 1993;17:78–83.
34. Bajzar L, Manuel R, Nesheim M. Purification and characterization of TAFI, a thrombin activatable fibrinolysis inhibitor. J Biol Chem 1995;270:14477–84.
35. Hendriks D, Wang W, Scharpe S, et al. Purification and characterization of a new arginine carboxypeptidase in human serum. Biochim Biophys Acta 1990;1034: 86–92.
36. Wang W, Hendriks DF, Scharpe S. Carboxypeptidase U, a plasma carboxypeptidase with high affinity for plasminogen. J Biol Chem 1994;269: 15937–44.
37. Sakharov D, Plow EF, Rijken DC. On the mechanism of the antifibrinolytic activity of plasma carboxypeptidase B. J Biol Chem 1997;272:14477–82.
38. Wang W, Boffa M, Bajzar L, et al. A study on the mechanism of activated thrombin-activatable fibrinolysis inhibitor. J Biol Chem 1998;273:27176–81.
39. Van Thiel DH, George M, Fareed J. Low levels of thrombin activatable fibrinolysis inhibitor (TAFI) in patients with chronic liver disease. Thromb Haemost 2001;85: 667–70.
40. Lisman T, Leebek FW, Mosnier LO, et al. Thrombin activatable fibrinolysis inhibitor deficiency in cirrhosis is not associated with increased plasma fibrinolysis. Gastroenterology 2001;121:131–9.
41. Colucci M, Binetti BM, Branca MG, et al. Deficiency of thrombin activatable fibrinolysis inhibitor in cirrhosis is associated with increased plasma fibrinolysis. Hepatology 2003;38:230–7.
42. Aytac S, Turkay C, Bavbek N, et al. Hemostasis and global fibrinolytic capacity in chronic liver disease. Blood Coagul Fibrinolysis 2007;18:623–6.
43. Thalheimer U, Triantos CK, Samonakis DN, et al. Infection, coagulation and variceal bleeding in cirrhosis. Gut 2005;54:556–63.
44. Agarwal S, Joyner KA, Swaim MW. Ascites fluid as a possible origin for hyperfibrinolysis in advanced liver disease. Am J Gastroenterol 2000;95: 3218–24.

45. Amitrano L, Guardascione MA, Brancaccio V, et al. Coagulation disorders in liver disease. Semin Liver Dis 2002;22:83–96.
46. Carr JM. Disseminated intravascular coagulation in cirrhosis. Hepatology 1989; 10:103–10.
47. Kemkes-Matthes B, Bleyl H, Matthes KJ. Coagulation activation in liver diseases. Thromb Res 1991;64:253–61.
48. Ben-Ari Z, Osman E, Ra Hutton, et al. Disseminated intravascular coagulation in liver cirrhosis: fact or fiction? Am J Gastroenterol 1999;94:2977–82.
49. Senzolo M, Burra P, Cholongitas E, et al. New insights into the coagulopathy of liver disease and liver transplantation. World J Gastroenterol 2006;12:7725–36.
50. Joist JH. AICF and DIC in liver cirrhosis: expressions of a hypercoagulable state. Am J Gastroenterol 1999;94:2801–3.
51. Tripodi A, Salerno F, Chantarangkul V, et al. Evidence of normal thrombin generation in cirrhosis despite abnormal conventional coagulation tests. Hepatology 2005;41:553–8.
52. Liehr H. Endotoxins and the pathogenesis of hepatic and gastrointestinal diseases. Internal Medicine and Pediatrics 1982;48:117–93.
53. Saliola M, Lorenzet R, Ferro D, et al. Enhanced expression of monocyte tissue factor in patients with liver cirrhosis. Gut 1998;43:428–32.
54. Violi F, Ferro D, Basili S, et al. Association between low-grade disseminated intravascular coagulation and endotoxemia in patients with liver cirrhosis. Gastroenterology 1995;109:531–9.
55. Garcia-Tsao G, Sanyal AJ, Grace ND, et al. Prevention and management of gastroesophageal varices and variceal hemorrhage in cirrhosis. Hepatology 2007; 46:922–38.
56. The North Italian Endoscopic Club for the Study and Treatment of Esophageal Varices. Prediction of the first variceal hemorrhage in patients with cirrhosis of the liver and esophageal varices. A prospective multicenter study. N Engl J Med 1988;319:983–9.
57. El Serag HB, Everhart JE. Improved survival after variceal hemorrhage over an 11-year period in the Department of Veterans Affairs. Am J Gastroenterol 2000; 95:3566–73.
58. D'Amico G, De Franchis R. Upper digestive bleeding in cirrhosis. Post-therapeutic outcome and prognostic indicators. Hepatology 2003;38:599–612.
59. Carbonell N, Pauwels A, Serfaty L, et al. Improved survival after variceal bleeding in patients with cirrhosis over the past two decades. Hepatology 2004;40: 652–9.
60. D'Amico G, Pagliaro L, Bosch J. Pharmacological treatment of portal hypertension: an evidence-based approach. Semin Liver Dis 1999;19:475–505.
61. Bosch J, Garcia-Pagan JC. Prevention of variceal rebleeding. Lancet 2003;361: 952–4.
62. Escorsell A, Bordas JM, Castaneda B, et al. Predictive value of the variceal pressure response to continued pharmacological therapy in patients with cirrhosis and portal hypertension. Hepatology 2000;31:1061–7.
63. Dell'Era A, Bosch J. The relevance of portal pressure and other risk factors in acute gastro-oesophageal variceal bleeding. Aliment Pharmacol Ther 2004; 20(Suppl 3):8–15.
64. Reverter JC. Abnormal hemostasis tests and bleeding in chronic liver disease: are they related? Yes. J.Thromb Haemost 2006;4:717–20.
65. Mannucci PM. Abnormal hemostasis tests and bleeding in chronic liver disease: are they related? No. J Thromb Haemost 2006;4:721–3.

66. Hedner U, Erhardtsen E. Hemostatic disorders in liver diseases. In: Schiff ER, Sorrell MF, Maddrey WC, editors. Schiff's diseases of the liver. Philadelphia: Lippincott Williams & Wilkins; 2003. p. 625–36.
67. Bosch J, D'Amico G, Garcia-Pagan JC. Portal hypertension. In: Schiff ER, Sorrell MF, Maddrey WC, editors. Schiff's diseases of the liver. Philadelphia: Lippincott Williams & Wilkins; 2003. p. 429–86.
68. Francis RB, Feinstein DI. Clinical significance of accelerated fibrinolysis in liver disease. Hemostasis 1984;14:460–5.
69. Bertaglia E, Belmonte P, Vertolli V, et al. Bleeding in cirrhotic patients: a precipitating factor due to intravascular coagulation or to hepatic failure? Hemostasis 1983; 13:328–34.
70. Violi F, Ferro D, Basili S, et al. Hyperfibrinolysis increases the risk of gastrointestinal hemorrhage in patients with advanced cirrhosis. Hepatology 1992;15:672–6.
71. Violi F, Basili S, Ferro D, et al. Association between high values of D-dimer and tissue-plasminogen activator activity and first gastrointestinal bleeding in cirrhotic patients. Thromb Haemost 1996;76:177–83.
72. Marder VJ, Sherry S. Thrombolytic therapy: current status. N Engl J Med 1988; 318:1585–95.
73. Stricker RB, Wong D, Shin DT, et al. Activation of plasminogen by tissue plasminogen activator on normal and thromboplastinic platelets: effects on surface proteins and platelet aggregation. Blood 1986;68:275–80.
74. Adelman B, Michelson AD, Greenberg J, et al. Proteolysis of platelet glycoprotein Ib by plasmin is facilitated by plasmin lysine-binding regions. Blood 1986;68:1280–4.
75. Loscalzo J, Vaughan DE. Tissue plasminogen activator promotes platelet disaggregation in plasma. J Commun Inq 1987;79:1749–55.
76. Bosch J, Reverter JC. The coagulopathy of cirrhosis: myth or reality? Hepatology 2005;41:434–5.
77. Massicotte L, Sassine MP, Lenis S, et al. Transfusion predictors in liver transplant. Anesth Analg 2004;98:1245–51.
78. Porte J. Coagulation and fibrinolysis in orthotopic liver transplantation: current views and insight. Semin Thromb Hemost 2003;19:191–8.
79. Hambleton J, Leung LL, Levi M. Coagulation: consultative hemostasis. Hematology Am Soc Hematol Educ Program 2002;10:335–52.
80. Homatas J, Wasantapruek S, Von Kaulla E, et al. Clotting abnormalities following orthotopic and heterotopic transplantation of marginally preserved pig livers. Acta Hepatosplenol 1971;18:14–26.
81. Richards EM, Alexander GJ, Calne RY, et al. Thrombocytopenia following liver transplantation is associated with platelet consumption and thrombin generation. Br J Haematol 1997;98:315–21.
82. Koh MB, Hunt BJ. The management of perioperative bleeding. Blood Rev 2003; 17:179–85.
83. Boylan JF, Klinck JR, Sandler AN, et al. Tranexamic acid reduces blood loss, transfusion requirements, and coagulation factor use in primary orthotopic liver transplantation. Anesthesiology 1996;85:1043–8.
84. Dalmau A, Sabaté A, Koo M, et al. The prophylactic use of tranexamic acid and aprotinin in orthotopic liver transplantation: a comparative study. Liver Transpl 2004;10:279–84.
85. Mannucci PM. Hemostatic drugs. N Engl J Med 1998;339:245–53.
86. Porte RJ, Molenaar IQ, Begliomini B, et al. Aprotinin and transfusion requirements in orthotopic liver transplantation: a multicentre randomised double-blind study. EMSALT Study Group. Lancet 2000;355:1303–9.

87. Molenaar IQ, Warnaar N, Groen H, et al. Efficacy and safety of antifibrinolytic drugs in liver transplantation: a systematic review and meta-analysis. Am J Transplant 2007;7:185–94.

88. Warnaar N, Mallett SV, de Boer MT, et al. The impact of aprotinin on renal function after liver transplantation: an analysis of 1,043 patients. Am J Transplant 2007;7:2378–87.

Superimposed Coagulopathic Conditions in Cirrhosis: Infection and Endogenous Heparinoids, Renal Failure, and Endothelial Dysfunction

Jasper H. Smalberg, MSc[a], Frank W.G. Leebeek, MD, PhD[a,b,*]

KEYWORDS

- Cirrhosis • Hemostasis • Infection
- Heparinoids • Renal failure • Endothelial dysfunction

Liver failure is accompanied by multiple changes in the hemostatic system.[1] These changes are mainly caused by a reduced synthesis of coagulation factors and altered clearance of activated coagulation factors. In addition, hyperfibrinolysis and thrombocytopenia are frequently encountered.[1] In this article, the authors discuss three additional pathophysiologic mechanisms that influence the coagulation system in patients who have liver disease. First, they discuss the influence of infections and endogenous heparinoids (see the related article elsewhere in this issue). Second, they discuss renal failure, a condition that is frequently encountered in patients who have liver cirrhosis. Finally, the dysfunction of the endothelial system is reviewed, including testing of endothelial function in liver disease.

[a] Department of Hematology, Erasmus University Medical Center, Rotterdam, The Netherlands
[b] The Netherlands Organisation for Scientific Research (NWO), Den Haag, The Netherlands
* Department of Hematology, Erasmus University Medical Center, Room L-435, P.O. Box 2040, 3000 GD Rotterdam, The Netherlands.
E-mail address: f.leebeek@erasmusmc.nl (F.W.G. Leebeek).

Clin Liver Dis 13 (2009) 33–42
doi:10.1016/j.cld.2008.09.006
1089-3261/08/$ – see front matter © 2009 Elsevier Inc. All rights reserved.

liver.theclinics.com

INFECTION AND ENDOGENOUS HEPARINOIDS

Bacterial infections are an important and frequently occurring coexisting problem in cirrhotic patients that is related to the degree of liver dysfunction.[2] They are reported in up to 47% of hospitalized cirrhotic patients[3] and result in increased mortality.[4] Bacterial infections have been reported in 35% to 66% of cirrhotic patients with gastrointestinal bleeding,[5] and infection is an independent risk factor for early rebleeding within 5 days of admission for variceal bleeding.[6,7] Furthermore, spontaneous bacterial peritonitis commonly precedes variceal bleeding[8] and recent evidence shows that prophylactic antibiotic therapy prevents early rebleeding.[9,10] This evidence illustrates the pivotal role of bacterial infections in the cause of variceal bleeding in patients who have liver cirrhosis.[11]

Endotoxemia is frequently found in cirrhotic patients,[12] originating from bacteria translocated from the bowel,[11] even in the absence of any signs of sepsis. Goulis and colleagues[13] postulated the role of bacterial infections through subsequent release of endotoxins in the systemic circulation as critical for triggering variceal bleeding through two distinct pathways. First, endotoxins lead to an increase in portal pressure by contracting hepatic stellate cells through the induction of endothelin.[14] Second, the release of nitric oxide (NO)[15–17] and prostacyclin[18,19] inhibits platelet aggregation.

Indeed, infection may lead to abnormalities in coagulation through multiple pathways. Sepsis can cause impairment of platelet aggregation, and production of cytokines in bacterial infections may lead to activation of clotting factors and fibrinolysis.[11] Here, the authors focus on the role of endogenous heparinoids. Heparinoids, both exogenous and endogenous, are cleared by the liver, and elevated levels have been reported in cirrhotic patients.[20] The influence of heparin-like substances is difficult to monitor in patients who have liver cirrhosis. Thromboelastography (TEG) is a quick and reliable method to assess clot formation and lysis and allows detection of heparin-like substances.[21] Using TEG, 20 cirrhotic patients were shown to exhibit worsening TEG parameters the day before rebleeding.[22] The same group demonstrated that bacterial infections significantly impair hemostasis in patients who have decompensated cirrhosis, also using TEG.[23] Montalto and colleagues[24] found a significant heparin activity using heparinase I–modified TEG in 28 of 30 cirrhotic patients, but none in those not infected, whereas other coagulation parameters were not altered. In a subsequent study, this heparin activity was found to be associated with anti–activated factor X concentrations in many patients.[25] Furthermore, the presence of endogenous heparinoids in cirrhotic patients who had acute variceal bleeding was demonstrated, which could contribute to failure to control acute bleeding and early rebleeding.[26] As a possible source for these endogenous heparinoids, it has been postulated that endotoxins and inflammation due to infection can release heparinoids from the endothelium and mast cells in a dose-dependent manner; in addition, endothelial cells are able to produce tissue-plasminogen activator, which induces fibrinolysis.[24]

Heparin and heparan sulfate belong to the family of glycosaminoglycans, which are heteropolysaccharides, including hyaluronic acid, chondroitin, dermatome sulfate, and keratan sulfate. Recently, it has been shown that heparinase I–modified TEG detects the activity of not only heparan sulfate but also dermatan sulfate, which indicates that both of these glycosaminoglycans could be responsible for the endogenous heparinoid effect.[27] However, evidence suggests that heparan sulfate, which is specifically cleaved by heparinase III–modified TEG, is the most important heparinoid responsible for the heparin-like effect.[28]

It can be concluded that the role of infection is well established in variceal bleeding in cirrhotic patients. Consequently, prophylactic antibiotics decrease the rate of bleeding. Therapeutic implications concerning the endogenous heparinoids in patients who have liver cirrhosis have not yet been identified.

RENAL FAILURE COAGULOPATHY IN CIRRHOSIS

Renal failure occurs frequently in patients who have liver cirrhosis.[29] Patients who have renal failure are at increased risk for bleeding complications.[30] Although the pathophysiology of this hemostatic dysfunction has not yet been fully elucidated, it appears to be multifactorial. Platelets play a pivotal role in the hemorrhagic tendencies in uremic patients.[30]

Platelet dysfunction occurs as a result of intrinsic platelet abnormalities and impaired platelet–vessel wall interaction.[31,32] Abnormalities of platelet alpha-granules with lower than normal content of ADP and serotonin[33,34] and defective arachidonic acid metabolism leading to decreased platelet thromboxane A2 generation have been reported in uremic patients.[35] Furthermore, functional and biochemical alterations of the platelet cytoskeleton in uremia were found.[36] Uremic platelets have a defective interaction with vessel subendothelium,[37] which may, in part, result from intrinsic dysfunction of glycoprotein GpIIb-IIIa, a platelet membrane glycoprotein that plays a major role in platelet aggregation and adhesion through its interaction with fibrinogen and von Willebrand factor (vWF).[33,38–40] Other causes of platelet dysfunction and impaired vessel wall interaction in uremia are discussed in more detail elsewhere in this issue.[30,41,42]

The potential role of uremic toxins and the vessel wall in uremic bleeding has also been extensively investigated. NO is a potent modulator of vascular tone that inhibits platelet adhesion to the endothelium[16] and platelet aggregation.[43] Studies in uremic patients have shown that platelet NO synthesis is increased and that uremic plasma stimulates NO production by cultured endothelial cells.[44] The increase in NO synthesis has been related to elevated levels of guanidinosuccinic acid, a uremic toxin that stimulates NO production in this setting.[30]

Anemia is common in uremic patients and is an important clinical risk factor for bleeding complications: the decreased number of red cells may rheologically reduce physical platelet interactions with the vessel wall and metabolically reduce platelet function.[42] Raising the hematocrit to 30% by red blood cell transfusions reduces the bleeding time in many patients, occasionally to a normal level.[45,46] Elevation of hematocrit can also be achieved by administrating recombinant human erythropoietin, which improves primary hemostasis through an increase of red cell mass but also through enhanced platelet aggregation and increased platelet adhesion to the endothelium, which is independent of the hematocrit rise.[47–50]

Hemodialysis also has a favorable impact on bleeding complications in uremic patients but may only partially correct platelet dysfunction.[51–54] In fact, the hemodialysis process itself may contribute to bleeding through the continuous platelet activation induced by the interaction between blood and artificial surfaces.[55]

Platelet transfusion is not effective in managing bleeding complications because uremic plasma elicits changes in function of platelets from normal donors.[42] Uremic plasma has been shown to inhibit platelet adhesion to inverted, de-endothelialized human umbilical cord artery segments, whereas uremic platelets adhere normally in the presence of normal plasma.[56] Therefore, rationale does not exist for platelet transfusion, which is sometimes used in interventions, such as dialysis line placement, to eliminate temporarily the bleeding tendency in uremic patients. Instead, current treatment modalities for uremic bleeding include erythropoietin, desmopressin, and estrogens, which have reduced bleeding complications.[42,57]

Although renal failure has classically been associated with a bleeding tendency, thrombotic events are also common among patients who have end-stage renal disease.[58] Various prothrombotic factors have been demonstrated in these patients. Elevated rates of thrombotic complications are thought to emerge as the bleeding tendency is better controlled.[59]

ENDOTHELIAL FUNCTION IN CIRRHOSIS

In recent years, the role of endothelial function in vascular health and disease has been studied extensively. The endothelium not only serves as a barrier between blood and the vessel wall but also plays an important role in hemostasis, vessel tone regulation, vascular homeostasis, and inflammatory processes. In response to various mechanical and chemical stimuli, endothelial cells secrete a wide array of substances that mediate these functions.[60–63] Endothelial dysfunction results in a loss of balance between prothrombotic and antithrombotic factors, vasoconstrictors and vasodilators, growth-promoting and growth-inhibiting factors, and proatherogenic and antiatherogenic factors,[62] and is now recognized as an essential part of the pathogenesis of several conditions, such as coronary artery disease[64,65] and microvascular complications in type 2 diabetes.[66]

Portal hypertension is primarily caused by increased resistance to portal blood flow, which, in cirrhosis, is mainly determined by morphologic changes.[67] However, substantial evidence shows that this is aggravated by a dynamic component, in which endothelial dysfunction plays a central role. Endothelial dysfunction causes an imbalance between the vasodilator and vasoconstrictor forces, affecting the vascular tone of the circulation on two distinct anatomic levels: the arteries of the intrahepatic microcirculation and the arteries of the splanchnic circulation.

Sinusoidal endothelial cells (SECs) play a central role in mediating intrahepatic vascular resistance by producing and releasing vasoactive substances.[68] A cirrhotic liver cannot accommodate the increased portal blood flow caused by postprandial hyperemia, resulting in an abrupt increase in portal pressure.[69] Such repeated increases are considered to be an important factor in progressive dilatation of varices in cirrhosis.[67] In addition, endothelial dysfunction in the hepatic vascular bed is characterized by a defective vasodilatory response to acetylcholine and insufficient NO production by endothelial NO synthase (eNOS).[70–72] Increased thromboxane A production in SECs has also been shown to contribute to increased intrahepatic resistance in cirrhosis.[73,74] Thus, SEC dysfunction impairs the endothelium-dependent dilatation of the intrahepatic liver microcirculation, resulting in increased intrahepatic vascular resistance and portal hypertension.

SEC dysfunction is an early event in the pathogenesis of cirrhosis[75] and is considered the primary event that leads to portal hypertension and the subsequent arterial splanchnic and systemic vasodilatation.[68] In contrast to the hypoactive SECs, an increased production of NO is observed in the arteries of the splanchnic and systemic circulation in cirrhosis and other conditions that lead to portal hypertension.[76] This increase in NO leads to an increased endothelium-dependent dilatation and precedes the so-called "hyperdynamic circulatory syndrome."[76–78] Several complications of liver cirrhosis, such as variceal bleeding, ascites, hepatorenal syndrome, and hepatopulmonary syndrome, are closely related to the presence of these hemodynamic alterations.[77]

Several clinical tests that evaluate endothelial function have been developed, mostly in relation to cardiovascular diseases.[79] Although clinical assessment of endothelial function tests in liver cirrhosis has received less attention, several promising markers of endothelial function in cirrhotic patients have been described. NO, its metabolites, and second messengers (cyclic GMP) are theoretically the clearest and most direct markers. Although assessment of vascular NO level is indicative of endothelial dysfunction in cirrhosis,[68] it is not yet widely used in clinical assessment of endothelial function. Interpretation of these measurements is often difficult and not always representative of endothelial NO production.[80] The procoagulant consequences of endothelial activation can be measured as a change in the balance of tissue-type plasminogen activator and plasminogen-activator inhibitor 1.[81] A shift in this balance, related to the extent of cirrhosis, has been reported.[82,83]

Furthermore, vWF is released into the circulation by activated endothelial cells and is easy to measure. Highly elevated levels of vWF in cirrhosis have been reported, which were strongly related to the severity of the disease.[84,85] Moreover, vWF levels were significantly correlated with NO production, as evaluated by nitrite and nitrate levels.[86] Endothelial cell activation leads to increased expression of inflammatory cytokines and adhesion molecules. Serum levels of intercellular adhesion molecule-1 are increased in cirrhosis[87] and are reported to be of prognostic relevance in patients who have liver cirrhosis.[88] Finally, substantial evidence exists for strongly elevated endothelin-1 levels in cirrhosis,[89] which may also be considered as an index for endothelial function.[61] To conclude, endothelial dysfunction testing appears promising for clinical research and should be evaluated in more detail for its clinical use.

Box 1
Mechanisms of superimposed conditions in liver cirrhosis leading to coagulopathic conditions

Bacterial infections/endotoxins

    Hemostatic imbalance

        Reduced platelet aggregation

        Activation clotting factors

        Hyperfibrinolysis

        Endogenous heparinoids

    Increased portal pressure (endothelin), predisposing to variceal bleeding

Renal failure

    Platelet abnormalities

    Impaired platelet–vessel wall interactions

    Anemia

    Abnormal NO production

    Others, such as drugs and comorbidity

Endothelial dysfunction

    Imbalance vasoconstrictors and vasodilators

    Intrahepatic vasoconstriction → increase of portal pressure

    Systemic vasodilatation → precedes hyperdynamic circulatory syndrome

SUMMARY

In this article, the authors discussed three superimposed coagulopathic conditions in patients who have liver cirrhosis, as summarized in **Box 1**. The pivotal role of infection in variceal bleeding is well established, and, among other things, it leads to abnormalities in coagulation. One of the pathways through which this occurs is shown to depend on endogenous heparinoids. Furthermore, renal failure may contribute to hemostatic imbalance in cirrhotic patients through so-called "uremic bleeding." Multifactorial platelet defects play a central role in the cause of uremic bleeding. Current treatment options include erythropoietin, desmopressin, and estrogens, which have been shown to reduce bleeding complications in renal failure. Finally, the authors discussed endothelial dysfunction, which is shown to play an important role in the development of portal hypertension in patients who have cirrhosis. Several promising markers of endothelial function in cirrhotic patients have recently become available and should be evaluated in more detail for their clinical use.

REFERENCES

1. Lisman T, Leebeek FW, de Groot PG. Haemostatic abnormalities in patients with liver disease. J Hepatol 2002;37(2):280–7.
2. Borzio M, Salerno F, Piantoni L, et al. Bacterial infection in patients with advanced cirrhosis: a multicentre prospective study. Dig Liver Dis 2001;33(1):41–8.
3. Caly WR, Strauss E. A prospective study of bacterial infections in patients with cirrhosis. J Hepatol 1993;18(3):353–8.
4. Rimola A, Soto R, Bory F, et al. Reticuloendothelial system phagocytic activity in cirrhosis and its relation to bacterial infections and prognosis. Hepatology 1984; 4(1):53–8.
5. Bernard B, Grange JD, Khac EN, et al. Antibiotic prophylaxis for the prevention of bacterial infections in cirrhotic patients with gastrointestinal bleeding: a meta-analysis. Hepatology 1999;29(6):1655–61.
6. Bernard B, Cadranel JF, Valla D, et al. Prognostic significance of bacterial infection in bleeding cirrhotic patients: a prospective study. Gastroenterology 1995; 108(6):1828–34.
7. Goulis J, Armonis A, Patch D, et al. Bacterial infection is independently associated with failure to control bleeding in cirrhotic patients with gastrointestinal hemorrhage. Hepatology 1998;27(5):1207–12.
8. Bleichner G, Boulanger R, Squara P, et al. Frequency of infections in cirrhotic patients presenting with acute gastrointestinal haemorrhage. Br J Surg 1986;73(9): 724–6.
9. Hou MC, Lin HC, Liu TT, et al. Antibiotic prophylaxis after endoscopic therapy prevents rebleeding in acute variceal hemorrhage: a randomized trial. Hepatology 2004;39(3):746–53.
10. Jun CH, Park CH, Lee WS, et al. Antibiotic prophylaxis using third generation cephalosporins can reduce the risk of early rebleeding in the first acute gastroesophageal variceal hemorrhage: a prospective randomized study. J Korean Med Sci 2006;21(5):883–90.
11. Thalheimer U, Triantos CK, Samonakis DN, et al. Infection, coagulation, and variceal bleeding in cirrhosis. Gut 2005;54(4):556–63.
12. Lin RS, Lee FY, Lee SD, et al. Endotoxemia in patients with chronic liver diseases: relationship to severity of liver diseases, presence of esophageal varices, and hyperdynamic circulation. J Hepatol 1995;22(2):165–72.

13. Goulis J, Patch D, Burroughs AK. Bacterial infection in the pathogenesis of variceal bleeding. Lancet 1999;353(9147):139–42.
14. Pinzani M, Milani S, De Franco R, et al. Endothelin 1 is overexpressed in human cirrhotic liver and exerts multiple effects on activated hepatic stellate cells. Gastroenterology 1996;110(2):534–48.
15. Laffi G, Foschi M, Masini E, et al. Increased production of nitric oxide by neutrophils and monocytes from cirrhotic patients with ascites and hyperdynamic circulation. Hepatology 1995;22(6):1666–73.
16. Radomski MW, Palmer RM, Moncada S. Endogenous nitric oxide inhibits human platelet adhesion to vascular endothelium. Lancet 1987;2(8567):1057–8.
17. Riddell DR, Graham A, Owen JS. Apolipoprotein E inhibits platelet aggregation through the L-arginine:nitric oxide pathway. Implications for vascular disease. J Biol Chem 1997;272(1):89–95.
18. Gratton JP, Maurice MC, D'Orleans-Juste P. Characterization of endothelin receptors and endothelin-converting enzyme activity in the rabbit lung. J Cardiovasc Pharmacol 1995;26(Suppl 3):S88–90.
19. Vane JR, Botting RM. Pharmacodynamic profile of prostacyclin. Am J Cardiol 1995;75(3):3A–10A.
20. Teien AN. Heparin elimination in patients with liver cirrhosis. Thromb Haemost 1977;38(3):701–6.
21. Salooja N, Perry DJ. Thrombelastography. Blood Coagul Fibrinolysis 2001;12(5):327–37.
22. Chau TN, Chan YW, Patch D, et al. Thrombelastographic changes and early rebleeding in cirrhotic patients with variceal bleeding. Gut 1998;43(2):267–71.
23. Papatheodoridis GV, Patch D, Webster GJ, et al. Infection and hemostasis in decompensated cirrhosis: a prospective study using thrombelastography. Hepatology 1999;29(4):1085–90.
24. Montalto P, Vlachogiannakos J, Cox DJ, et al. Bacterial infection in cirrhosis impairs coagulation by a heparin effect: a prospective study. J Hepatol 2002;37(4):463–70.
25. Zambruni A, Thalheimer U, Coppell J, et al. Endogenous heparin-like activity detected by anti-Xa assay in infected cirrhotic and non-cirrhotic patients. Scand J Gastroenterol 2004;39(9):830–6.
26. Thalheimer U, Triantos C, Samonakis D, et al. Endogenous heparinoids in acute variceal bleeding. Gut 2005;54(2):310–1.
27. Senzolo M, Coppell J, Cholongitas E, et al. The effects of glycosaminoglycans on coagulation: a thromboelastographic study. Blood Coagul Fibrinolysis 2007;18(3):227–36.
28. Senzolo M, Cholangitas E, Riddell A, et al. Heparinase I, II and III modified thromboelastography for the detection of different glycosaminoglycans' effect in cirrhotics with bacterial infection. J Hepatol 2006;44(Suppl 2):S72.
29. Arroyo V, Gines P, Gerbes AL, et al. Definition and diagnostic criteria of refractory ascites and hepatorenal syndrome in cirrhosis. International Ascites Club. Hepatology 1996;23(1):164–76.
30. Noris M, Remuzzi G. Uremic bleeding: closing the circle after 30 years of controversies? Blood 1999;94(8):2569–74.
31. Livio M, Benigni A, Remuzzi G. Coagulation abnormalities in uremia. Semin Nephrol 1985;5(2):82–90.
32. Remuzzi G. Bleeding in renal failure. Lancet 1988;1(8596):1205–8.
33. Di Minno G, Cerbone A, Usberti M, et al. Platelet dysfunction in uremia. II. Correction by arachidonic acid of the impaired exposure of fibrinogen receptors by adenosine diphosphate or collagen. J Lab Clin Med 1986;108(3):246–52.

34. Eknoyan G, Brown CH 3rd. Biochemical abnormalities of platelets in renal failure. Evidence for decreased platelet serotonin, adenosine diphosphate and Mg-dependent adenosine triphosphatase. Am J Nephrol 1981;1(1):17–23.

35. Remuzzi G, Benigni A, Dodesini P, et al. Reduced platelet thromboxane formation in uremia. Evidence for a functional cyclooxygenase defect. J Clin Invest 1983; 71(3):762–8.

36. Escolar G, Diaz-Ricart M, Cases A, et al. Abnormal cytoskeletal assembly in platelets from uremic patients. Am J Pathol 1993;143(3):823–31.

37. Castillo R, Lozano T, Escolar G, et al. Defective platelet adhesion on vessel sub-endothelium in uremic patients. Blood 1986;68(2):337–42.

38. Benigni A, Boccardo P, Galbusera M, et al. Reversible activation defect of the platelet glycoprotein IIb-IIIa complex in patients with uremia. Am J Kidney Dis 1993;22(5):668–76.

39. Escolar G, Cases A, Bastida E, et al. Uremic platelets have a functional defect affecting the interaction of von Willebrand factor with glycoprotein IIb-IIIa. Blood 1990;76(7):1336–40.

40. Gawaz MP, Dobos G, Spath M, et al. Impaired function of platelet membrane glycoprotein IIb-IIIa in end-stage renal disease. J Am Soc Nephrol 1994;5(1):36–46.

41. Sohal AS, Gangji AS, Crowther MA, et al. Uremic bleeding: pathophysiology and clinical risk factors. Thromb Res 2006;118(3):417–22.

42. Weigert AL, Schafer AI. Uremic bleeding: pathogenesis and therapy. Am J Med Sci 1998;316(2):94–104.

43. Marietta M, Facchinetti F, Neri I, et al. L-arginine infusion decreases platelet aggregation through an intraplatelet nitric oxide release. Thromb Res 1997;88(2):229–35.

44. Noris M, Benigni A, Boccardo P, et al. Enhanced nitric oxide synthesis in uremia: implications for platelet dysfunction and dialysis hypotension. Kidney Int 1993; 44(2):445–50.

45. Fernandez F, Goudable C, Sie P, et al. Low haematocrit and prolonged bleeding time in uraemic patients: effect of red cell transfusions. Br J Haematol 1985;59(1): 139–48.

46. Livio M, Gotti E, Marchesi D, et al. Uraemic bleeding: role of anaemia and beneficial effect of red cell transfusions. Lancet 1982;2(8306):1013–5.

47. Cases A, Escolar G, Reverter JC, et al. Recombinant human erythropoietin treatment improves platelet function in uremic patients. Kidney Int 1992;42(3):668–72.

48. Fabris F, Cordiano I, Randi ML, et al. Effect of human recombinant erythropoietin on bleeding time, platelet number and function in children with end-stage renal disease maintained by haemodialysis. Pediatr Nephrol 1991;5(2):225–8.

49. Moia M, Mannucci PM, Vizzotto L, et al. Improvement in the haemostatic defect of uraemia after treatment with recombinant human erythropoietin. Lancet 1987; 2(8570):1227–9.

50. Van Geet C, Van Damme-Lombaerts R, Vanrusselt M, et al. Recombinant human erythropoietin increases blood pressure, platelet aggregability and platelet free calcium mobilisation in uraemic children: a possible link? Thromb Haemost 1990;64(1):7–10.

51. Di Minno G, Martinez J, McKean ML, et al. Platelet dysfunction in uremia. Multifaceted defect partially corrected by dialysis. Am J Med 1985;79(5):552–9.

52. Rabiner SF. The effect of dialysis on platelet function of patients with renal failure. Ann N Y Acad Sci 1972;201:234–42.

53. Remuzzi G, Livio M, Marchiaro G, et al. Bleeding in renal failure: altered platelet function in chronic uraemia only partially corrected by haemodialysis. Nephron 1978;22(4–6):347–53.

54. Stewart JH, Castaldi PA. Uraemic bleeding: a reversible platelet defect corrected by dialysis. Q J Med 1967;36(143):409–23.
55. Boccardo P, Remuzzi G, Galbusera M. Platelet dysfunction in renal failure. Semin Thromb Hemost 2004;30(5):579–89.
56. Zwaginga JJ, Ijsseldijk MJ, Beeser-Visser N, et al. High von Willebrand factor concentration compensates a relative adhesion defect in uremic blood. Blood 1990;75(7):1498–508.
57. Hedges SJ, Dehoney SB, Hooper JS, et al. Evidence-based treatment recommendations for uremic bleeding. Nat Clin Pract Nephrol 2007;3(3):138–53.
58. Casserly LF, Dember LM. Thrombosis in end-stage renal disease. Semin Dial 2003;16(3):245–56.
59. Escolar G, Diaz-Ricart M, Cases A. Uremic platelet dysfunction: past and present. Curr Hematol Rep 2005;4(5):359–67.
60. Caballero AE. Endothelial dysfunction in obesity and insulin resistance: a road to diabetes and heart disease. Obes Res 2003;11(11):1278–89.
61. Laffi G, Marra F. Complications of cirrhosis: is endothelium guilty? J Hepatol 1999; 30(3):532–5.
62. Quyyumi AA. Endothelial function in health and disease: new insights into the genesis of cardiovascular disease. Am J Med 1998;105(1A):32S–9S.
63. Racanelli V, Rehermann B. The liver as an immunological organ. Hepatology 2006;43(2 Suppl 1):S54–62.
64. Mano T, Masuyama T, Yamamoto K, et al. Endothelial dysfunction in the early stage of atherosclerosis precedes appearance of intimal lesions assessable with intravascular ultrasound. Am Heart J 1996;131(2):231–8.
65. Ross R. Atherosclerosis–an inflammatory disease. N Engl J Med 1999;340(2): 115–26.
66. Tooke JE. Microvascular function in human diabetes. A physiological perspective. Diabetes 1995;44(7):721–6.
67. Bosch J, Garcia-Pagan JC. Complications of cirrhosis. I. Portal hypertension. J Hepatol 2000;32(1 Suppl):141–56.
68. Iwakiri Y, Groszmann RJ. Vascular endothelial dysfunction in cirrhosis. J Hepatol 2007;46(5):927–34.
69. Bellis L, Berzigotti A, Abraldes JG, et al. Low doses of isosorbide mononitrate attenuate the postprandial increase in portal pressure in patients with cirrhosis. Hepatology 2003;37(2):378–84.
70. Gupta TK, Toruner M, Chung MK, et al. Endothelial dysfunction and decreased production of nitric oxide in the intrahepatic microcirculation of cirrhotic rats. Hepatology 1998;28(4):926–31.
71. Rockey DC, Chung JJ. Reduced nitric oxide production by endothelial cells in cirrhotic rat liver: endothelial dysfunction in portal hypertension. Gastroenterology 1998;114(2):344–51.
72. Sarela AI, Mihaimeed FM, Batten JJ, et al. Hepatic and splanchnic nitric oxide activity in patients with cirrhosis. Gut 1999;44(5):749–53.
73. Graupera M, Garcia-Pagan JC, Pares M, et al. Cyclooxygenase-1 inhibition corrects endothelial dysfunction in cirrhotic rat livers. J Hepatol 2003;39(4): 515–21.
74. Graupera M, March S, Engel P, et al. Sinusoidal endothelial COX-1-derived prostanoids modulate the hepatic vascular tone of cirrhotic rat livers. Am J Physiol Gastrointest Liver Physiol 2005;288(4):G763–70.
75. Braet F, Wisse E. Structural and functional aspects of liver sinusoidal endothelial cell fenestrae: a review. Comp Hepatol 2002;1(1):1.

76. Iwakiri Y, Groszmann RJ. The hyperdynamic circulation of chronic liver diseases: from the patient to the molecule. Hepatology 2006;43(2 Suppl 1):S121–31.
77. Groszmann RJ, Abraldes JG. Portal hypertension: from bedside to bench. J Clin Gastroenterol 2005;39(4 Suppl 2):S125–30.
78. Wiest R, Groszmann RJ. The paradox of nitric oxide in cirrhosis and portal hypertension: too much, not enough. Hepatology 2002;35(2):478–91.
79. Deanfield JE, Halcox JP, Rabelink TJ. Endothelial function and dysfunction: testing and clinical relevance. Circulation 2007;115(10):1285–95.
80. Vapaatalo H, Mervaala E. Clinically important factors influencing endothelial function. Med Sci Monit 2001;7(5):1075–85.
81. Vaughan DE. PAI-1 and atherothrombosis. J Thromb Haemost 2005;3(8): 1879–83.
82. Leebeek FW, Kluft C, Knot EA, et al. A shift in balance between profibrinolytic and antifibrinolytic factors causes enhanced fibrinolysis in cirrhosis. Gastroenterology 1991;101(5):1382–90.
83. Violi F, Ferro D, Quintarelli C, et al. Clotting abnormalities in chronic liver disease. Dig Dis 1992;10(3):162–72.
84. Ferro D, Quintarelli C, Lattuada A, et al. High plasma levels of von Willebrand factor as a marker of endothelial perturbation in cirrhosis: relationship to endotoxemia. Hepatology 1996;23(6):1377–83.
85. Lisman T, Bongers TN, Adelmeijer J, et al. Elevated levels of von Willebrand factor in cirrhosis support platelet adhesion despite reduced functional capacity. Hepatology 2006;44(1):53–61.
86. Albornoz L, Alvarez D, Otaso JC, et al. Von Willebrand factor could be an index of endothelial dysfunction in patients with cirrhosis: relationship to degree of liver failure and nitric oxide levels. J Hepatol 1999;30(3):451–5.
87. Bruno CM, Sciacca C, Cilio D, et al. Circulating adhesion molecules in patients with virus-related chronic diseases of the liver. World J Gastroenterol 2005; 11(29):4566–9.
88. Giron-Gonzalez JA, Martinez-Sierra C, Rodriguez-Ramos C, et al. Adhesion molecules as a prognostic marker of liver cirrhosis. Scand J Gastroenterol 2005; 40(2):217–24.
89. Mallat A, Lotersztajn S. Multiple hepatic functions of endothelin-1: physiopathological relevance. J Hepatol 1996;25(3):405–13.

Heparin-like Effect in Liver Disease and Liver Transplantation

M. Senzolo, MD, PhD[a], E. Cholongitas, MD[b], U. Thalheimer, MD, PhD[b],
Anne Riddell, PhD[c], S. Agarwal, MB, MS, FRCA[d], S. Mallett, MB, MS, FRCA[d],
C. Ferronato, MD[a], A.K. Burroughs, MBChB Hons, FRCP[b,*]

KEYWORDS
- Liver disease • Bleeding • Coagulation
- Heparinoids • Liver transplantation

The liver has key roles in blood coagulation in primary and secondary hemostasis.[1] It is the site of synthesis of all coagulation factors and their inhibitors, except von Willebrand factor.[2] Liver damage is commonly associated with impairment of coagulation, when liver function reserve is poor. These hemostatic abnormalities do not always lead to spontaneous bleeding. Recently, the generation of thrombin has been explored in vitro in stable patients who have cirrhosis, and found to be normal when the anticoagulation pathway was activated by the addition of thrombomodulin (see also the article by Tripodi in this issue). In this study, a resetting of the coagulation and anticoagulation system at a lower level was postulated, because in the presence of liver disease, procoagulant and anticoagulant pathways are affected in a parallel manner, thus maintaining hemostatic balance.[3] However, the in vitro technique has some drawbacks, the major ones being the exclusion of cellular components of blood, in particular, platelets, which were substituted by phospholipids.[3] Recently, however, the same investigators have shown that when the number of platelets was adjusted to correspond to whole-blood counts, patients who had cirrhosis generated significantly less thrombin than controls.[4] Indeed, patients who have cirrhosis do have an increased bleeding tendency.

This delicate hemostatic balance can be perturbed by numerous conditions, such as variceal bleeding, renal failure, or infection/sepsis, which may lead to worsening of coagulation status.

[a] Division of Gastroenterology, Department of Surgical and Gastroenterological Sciences, University Hospital of Padua, Via Giustiniani 2, 35136, Padova, Italy
[b] The Royal Free Sheila Sherlock Liver Centre and Department of Surgery, Royal Free Hospital, Pond Street, London NW3 2QG, UK
[c] Department of Heamophilia and Haemostasis, Royal Free Hospital, Pond Street, London NW3 2QG, UK
[d] Department of Anesthesia, Royal Free Hospital, Pond Street, London NW3 2QG, UK
* Corresponding author.
E-mail address: andrew.burroughs@royalfree.nhs.uk (A.K. Burroughs).

Clin Liver Dis 13 (2009) 43–53
doi:10.1016/j.cld.2008.09.004
1089-3261/08/$ – see front matter © 2009 Elsevier Inc. All rights reserved.

liver.theclinics.com

INFECTION, COAGULATION, AND HEPARIN-LIKE EFFECT

The overall cumulative incidence of infection in cirrhotic patients is estimated to be at least 30%,[5] and it is possibly associated with an increased risk for variceal bleeding;[6] moreover, infection is associated with early rebleeding and increased mortality.[7,8] Prophylactic antibiotic therapy has led to less early rebleeding and better control of bleeding, in two randomized studies.[9,10] Infection affects different sides of coagulation. Sepsis can cause impairment of platelet function, decreasing platelet number and aggregation because of increased nitric oxide (NO) production.[11] In addition, cytokines, in particular interleukin 6 and tumor necrosis factor-alfa, released during infection, can trigger a disseminated intravascular coagulation (DIC)-like picture with hyperfibrinolysis.[12] One study showed a strong association between fragment F1+2 and D-dimer with endotoxemia: these markers returned to normal after antibiotic therapy.[13] Another report recently showed decreased platelet count and levels of factor VII, X, V, and II, in cirrhotic patients and severe sepsis, suggesting consumptive coagulopathy,[14] whereas a further study found decreased activity of protein C, which is associated with increased fibrinolysis.[15]

Recently, the role of heparin-like substances has been studied in the worsening of coagulation in patients who have cirrhosis and bacterial infection. Twenty cirrhotic patients who experienced early rebleeding after variceal bleeding were studied prospectively and found to have worsening thromboelastography (TEG) parameters the day before rebleeding[16] compared with cirrhotics, who did not rebleed. This finding was not accompanied by different values of standard coagulation parameters, and the only difference between the two groups was the incidence of bacterial infection. This gave rise to a hypothesis that an increased amount of endogenous heparin-like substances could be responsible, in part, for the risk for bleeding in cirrhotics with varices and that occurrence this may be linked to the presence of infection. The role of infection in decompensated cirrhotics was further evaluated by Papatheodoridis and colleagues,[17] who showed that patients who had cirrhosis and infection had worse TEG parameters compared with noninfected patients and that these parameters worsened if the infection did not resolve. The role of heparinoids in the coagulopathy of patients who have cirrhosis and infection was then investigated in a further study, using heparinase I–modified TEG. Heparinase I is produced by *Flavobacterium heparinum* and, unlike protamine, it antagonizes the effects of heparin-like substances without, itself, affecting TEG variables.[18,19]

In the study by Montalto and colleagues,[20] 28 of 30 infected cirrhotics showed a heparin-like effect (HLE) in the TEG trace compared with none of the noninfected patients (**Fig. 1**). This apparent HLE resolved in 8 cirrhotics re-evaluated after the resolution of infection, which supported a possible role of endogenous heparinoids in the bleeding tendency of patients who have cirrhosis. Moreover, an effect of endogenous heparinoids was not found in infected patients who did not have liver disease, probably because the normal liver is able to clear them. The presence of heparin-like substances detected by TEG during infection in cirrhosis is associated, in some, with increased anti–activated factor X (Xa) activity, which correlates with the TEG parameters (*r* time) when corrected by heparinase I.[21] The anti-Xa activity seen in infected cirrhotic patients can be explained by the increased amount of heparin-like substances, which are able to increase antithrombin activity and cannot be properly cleaved by the damaged liver.

Several possible mechanisms could lead to the presence of endogenous heparinoids and the anti-Xa activity induced by bacterial infections in patients who have liver cirrhosis and, possibly, also in noncirrhotic patients. NO production is enhanced by

A

Native

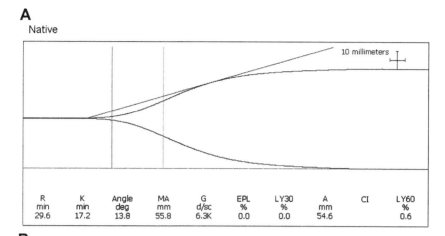

R min	K min	Angle deg	MA mm	G d/sc	EPL %	LY30 %	A mm	CI	LY60 %
29.6	17.2	13.8	55.8	6.3K	0.0	0.0	54.6		0.6

B

Heparinase I modified TEG

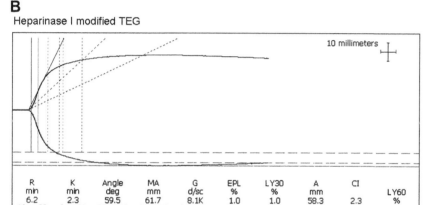

R min	K min	Angle deg	MA mm	G d/sc	EPL %	LY30 %	A mm	CI	LY60 %
6.2	2.3	59.5	61.7	8.1K	1.0	1.0	58.3	2.3	*2.3*
16 — 23	6 — 11	22 — 38	47 — 58	4.2K — 6.1K	0 — 15	0 — 8		-3 — 3	

Fig. 1. Presence of heparin-like effect (HLE) in a patient who had cirrhosis and peritoneal infection. Native TEG (*A*) and heparinase I–TEG (*B*) on sample collected at the onset of spontaneous bacterial peritonitis in a patient who had liver cirrhosis. A significant HLE was found; the slowed rate of coagulation in *A* compared with *B* is shown by the decrease in slope (lower angle of separation). Treatment of the sample in *B* with heparinases increases the rate of coagulation, thus sampling the presence of heparin-like substances.

endotoxins and cytokines, and plasma-related products, nitrites, and nitrates correlate with the level of endotoxemia in patients who have cirrhosis.[22] NO has been recently shown by Nielsen[23] to affect the blood coagulation as assessed by TEG (*r* time and *a* angle) in rabbits, probably by the direct inhibition of the serine proteases, such as clotting factor X, by way of the nitrosylation of sulfhydryl groups critical for their function. With this mechanism, no endogenous heparin-like substances would be involved, and one should not find any amelioration in TEG parameters with heparinase I. Another mechanism could be that, during sepsis, the liver is exposed to a neutrophil-mediated injury involving hepatocytes and endothelial cells,[24] which could release heparin-like substances into the systemic circulation, analogous to what happens during suramin treatment in patients who have metastatic liver disease.[25] The liver contains abundant parenchymal glycosaminoglycans (GAGs) deposits, heparan sulfate being one of the most plentiful constituents.[26] Additionally, the extracellular proteases produced by leukocytes during bacterial infections[27] could unmask circulating GAGs from their binding with plasmatic peptidic ligands, increasing their availability and activity.[28] The anticoagulant activity of circulating GAGs in experimental settings only appears after exhaustive proteolytic digestion of plasma.[28] Lastly, as previously suggested by the authors' group, bacterial infections could lead to mast cell activation, with the consequent release in the circulation of heparin and other mediators with anticoagulant activity.[20]

All four mechanisms could potentially be involved simultaneously and in different proportions, thus leading to a dynamic process that could account for the individual variability of the anticoagulant effects of infections.

Endogenous heparinoids are GAGs that are constituents of the vessels and are both synthesized and linked to the endothelial wall, being natural anticoagulants. GAGs are a group of complex polysaccharides, the main ones being heparin and heparan sulfate, but they also include hyaluronan, chondroitin sulfate, dermatan sulfate, and keratin sulfate.[29]

The mixture of heparinoids, Danaparoid, used therapeutically in surgery in patients who have an adverse reaction to heparin, is a mixture of heparan, dermatan, and chondroitin sulfate; it has been shown to inhibit TEG trace. Recently, heparinase I–modified TEG has been shown to be more effective in correcting the TEG trace to normal compared with protamine sulfate, in blood that had Danaparoid added to it.[30] Heparinase I is able specifically to cleave heparin[31] and, less effectively, heparan monosulfate (72% less effective);[32] it has been not shown to be able to detect dermatan sulfate activity. Therefore, it is still not clear which GAG is responsible for the HLE detected in cirrhotic patients by TEG and anti-Xa activity.

Heparin-like Effect and Liver Transplant

Liver transplant is frequently complicated by severe coagulopathy, particularly after reperfusion of the grafted liver. The causes of marked deterioration in coagulation that accompanies reperfusion have been identified as hyperfibrinolysis, DIC, platelet activation, trapping of platelets in the graft, and the presence of HLE.[33] The TEG has been shown to be a useful monitor of coagulation abnormalities during liver transplant, providing a rational approach for transfusion of blood components.[34] Moreover, heparinase I–modified TEG does detect the presence of heparin-like substances in patients undergoing liver transplant before and after reperfusion, described for the first time during human liver transplant by Kang and colleagues[33] in 1985. The HLE subsequently resolved spontaneously in most patients within 1 to 2 hours of reperfusion, without any treatment. Bakker and colleagues,[35] using protamine titrated in vitro, demonstrated an HLE in all of 15 recipients when heparin was infused to the venous system of the donor liver before harvesting, and in none of the residual 5 patients in which this procedure was not performed. This finding suggested that heparin bound to the donor liver endothelium could be subsequently flushed into the systemic circulation of the recipient after reperfusion. However, an endogenous source of heparinoids was also postulated, because evidence of heparin-like activity was reported after reperfusion even in the absence of heparin infusion in the donor liver.[35] In addition, two cases have been reported of reversal of similar TEG abnormalities, prolonged kaolin cephalin clotting time, and cessation of oozing after administration of protamine, 50 mg, during reperfusion phase.[36]

Before the advent of heparinase-coated cups in TEG, the prevalence of HLE in patients undergoing liver transplant was reported to be between 25% and 95% of cases.[37,38] In the last 10 years, three large series using heparinase I–modified TEG have reported the prevalence of HLE among patients undergoing liver transplant.[35,39–42] The most recent, which studied a larger number of 211 patients, is in press.[43] The relevance of HLE after reperfusion ranged from 75% to 93% of patients in the other two studies, giving only mean values and not reporting the prevalence.[39,40] In one study, the appearance of HLE was correlated with increased blood requirements only when abnormal coagulation tests were present,[42] although Agarwal and colleagues[43] did not find this association.

Two studies[40,43] showed HLE before incision (**Table 1**). The larger study showed a prevalence of 30%, 6% being severe (ie, a correction of the TEG by heparinase by more than 80%). A higher prevalence of HLE is seen in patients who have acute liver failure[44] or primary nonfunction of the liver graft and in patients urgently listed for retransplant,[43] but the cause is still unknown. Kang and colleagues,[33] Pivalizza and colleagues,[39] and Harding and colleagues,[42] all used protamine sulfate to antagonize the effects of endogenous heparinoids. Only one case report describes the use of protamine in an attempt to reduce oozing because of an appearance of a severe HLE after reperfusion,[36] but evidence for a therapeutic effect of reversing HLE has been little studied.

Thus, in liver transplantation, an exogenous source of heparin released after reperfusion exists, because of residual heparin bound to the endothelium of the donor vessels, as the donor liver is perfused with heparin before clamping. However, an endogenous source of heparinoids also exists because in some recipients they are present before incision, and, in addition, an increased release of heparinoids is thought to occur from activation of macrophages following the ischemia reperfusion injury. The presence of heparinoids is correlated with the severity of liver disease,[40,45] probably because of decreased cleavage by the liver of endogenous and exogenous heparin heparinoids.[42] The cause of liver disease does not seem to influence the presence and severity of HLE. Moreover, after experimental CCL4 cirrhosis in rats, levels of a highly sulfated heparinoid increased more than 10 fold, although the effect on coagulation has not been evaluated.[46] It is still unclear what the identity is of the endogenous heparinoids responsible for the HLE after reperfusion of the graft and, in some patients, throughout the liver transplant procedure.

THE EFFECT OF GLYCOSAMINOGLYCANS ON COAGULATION AND THEIR ACTIVITY IN LIVER DISEASE AND LIVER TRANSPLANT

The prime site of regulation of hemostasis is the surfaces of vascular endothelial cells, which have been known to possess anticoagulant properties.[47] These properties are particularly conspicuous in the microcirculation, with its high wall-surface-to-blood-volume

Table 1
Summary of the published studies reporting on heparin-like effect at different stages during liver transplant

Investigators	Number of Patients	HLE before Reperfusion	HLE after Reperfusion	Correlation with Blood Loss	Use of Protamine
Harding et al	55	NA	71%	Yes	Yes[a]
Pivalizza et al	26	No	100%	NA	NA
Kettner et al	72	100%	100%	NA	NA
Agarwal et al	211	31%	75%	No	No

Abbreviation: NA, not available.
[a] Only when associated with alterated standard laboratory test revealing an hypocoagulative status.

ratio. The ability of certain sulfated polysaccharides, GAGs, to interfere with blood co-agulation has been known for some time, as evidenced by the extensive clinical use of heparin as an antithrombotic agent. GAGs (heparinoids) are widely distributed in an-imal tissues and appear to be synthesized by virtually all types of cells, but are mainly constituents of the vessel wall and can be bound by the endothelium.[48] Endothelial cells synthesize heparan sulfate but are also able to bind other heparin-like sub-stances, such as dermatan and chondroitin sulfate.[28,49] All these GAGs have antico-agulation properties and help maintain coagulation hemostasis at the endothelial surface. Heparan sulfate is the most important GAG, but dermatan sulfate has recently been recognized to have important anticoagulation properties because it inactivates coagulation enzymes by binding with antithrombin.[50] Dermatan sulfate inhibits throm-bin generation by forming an inactive ternary complex with heparin cofactor II;[51] it has also been shown to be as effective as heparin in preventing postoperative thrombosis, and can be used as an alternative to heparin when heparin-induced thrombocytopenia occurs.[52]

Chondroitin 4 and 6 sulfate are mainly present in cartilage but are also constituents of the vessel wall and can be bound by endothelial cells.[28] They are not recognized to have an anticoagulative effect through thrombin inhibition.[53] Recently, however, such an effect has been demonstrated by a change in water content of arteriosclerotic pla-ques.[54] Furthermore, in its fucosylated form, chondroitin sulfate protects vessels from thrombosis and prevents shunt stenosis in experimental rats.[55]

The activity in vivo of Danaparoid (ie, a mixture of heparin, dermatan, and chondroi-tin sulfate) used therapeutically can only be evaluated by measuring anti-Xa activity. Therefore, recently, heparinase I–modified TEG has been evaluated to detect and monitor its effects in vitro, but a direct statistical correlation between the concentration of Danaparoid and its anticoagulation properties has not been demonstrated.[30] However, the effect of the component GAGs that constitute Danaparoid has not been evaluated. Senzolo and colleagues[56] recently demonstrated that heparinase I–modified TEG is able to detect not only the effect of heparan sulfate but also spe-cifically that of dermatan sulfate, a finding not documented previously. The inhibition of clotting by dermatan and heparan sulfate was fully reversed by heparinase I. Both these compounds inhibited thrombin formation, resulting in increased levels of anti-Xa activity, even if, as previously shown, a direct correlation between anti-Xa-activity and inhibition of clotting could not be shown. The above GAGs also produce their activity through an interaction with heparin cofactor II. Based on these findings, it can be hypothesized that potentially each and every GAG could be responsible for the HLE seen by heparinase I–modified TEG in patients who have cirrhosis and bacterial infection.[57]

Activity of endogenous GAGs has only been characterized in a few cases and mostly is attributed to heparan sulfate.[45,58–60] In one study, anticoagulation was as-cribed to a high-affinity heparin in a patient who had metastatic bladder carcinoma,[61] whereas in another, it was attributed to dermatan sulfate after suramin treatment, in a patient who had metastatic liver carcinoma.[25] Only one study, as yet not repeated, showed an increased heparan sulfate concentration in cirrhotic patients who had recent variceal bleeding compared with patients who had cirrhosis without bleeding and noncirrhotic patients who had bled.[45] The levels of heparan sulfate were higher in those who had more severe liver disease, suggesting an impaired capacity to elim-inate heparinoids in cirrhosis. Recently, the authors' group has used TEG with the addition of a new heparinase specific for cleaving only heparan sulfate,[62] which shows that the anticoagulant activity can be attributed to heparan sulfate in patients who have liver cirrhosis and bacterial infection.[63]

During liver transplant, exogenous heparin is responsible for most or part of the HLE seen after reperfusion, but identification of specific endogenous heparinoids throughout the different stages during liver transplantation have not been reported, with the exception of one study in a pediatric population by Mitchell and colleagues.[64] Fluctuating levels of heparan and dermatan sulfate at all time points during transplant and up to 3 weeks after the operation were found in all the pediatric patients.[64]

Therapeutic Implications

Prevention of infection during variceal bleeding is a well-defined treatment, recognized to be able to reduce rebleeding and mortality.[9,10] The effect of the treatment of infection may be due to the prevention of worsening portal hemodynamics but has been shown indirectly only by one study by Ruiz-del-Arbol and colleagues,[65] in which hepatic venous pressure gradient was higher with spontaneous bacterial peritonitis but did not always return to baseline with resolution of infection, but also of coagulation due to infection which appears deranged at TEG hours after the bleeding.[66]

Infusion of protamine sulfate has been attempted in a few studies aiming to revert the HLE seen after reperfusion in cirrhotic patients,[36] although its effect in reducing bleeding and blood unit requirement was not clearly demonstrated. Use of heparinase I in vivo (Neutralase) has been investigated recently to treat coagulopathy due to the release of exogenous heparin in patients undergoing coronary artery bypass, but it has been shown to worsen the outcome compared with standard protamine treatment.[67] Theoretically, the ability of heparinase I to cleave endogenous heparinoids more specifically than protamine could offer an advantage in patients who have demonstrable HLE due to endogenous GAGs such as in cirrhotics with infection or bleeding, but its clinical role has still to be formally investigated.

SUMMARY

Liver cirrhosis is characterized by impairment of primary and secondary hemostasis, but it is not clear how this is related to bleeding. This delicate hemostatic balance can be perturbed by numerous conditions, such as variceal bleeding, renal failure, or infection/sepsis, which may lead to worsening of the coagulation status. The role of endogenous heparinoids (GAGs) in the coagulopathy of patients who have liver cirrhosis has been demonstrated by the use of TEG with the addition of heparinase I in patients who had recent variceal bleeding and infection. This effect seems to be mediated by an anticoagulant activity similar to low weight molecular heparin. A decreased capacity of the cirrhotic liver to cleave heparin-like substances, together with an increased release of heparinoids by macrophages or hepatocytes or endothelium during sepsis, is the potential mechanism involved. The HLE has also been demonstrated to be part of the coagulopathy seen after reperfusion in patients who have cirrhosis and are undergoing liver transplant, with a prevalence ranging from 71% to 100%. However, the appearance of the HLE correlated with increased blood requirements only when abnormal coagulation tests were present. An exogenous source of heparin from the endothelium of the donor hepatic vessels can be demonstrated, although an endogenous source is also present because the HLE can be detected before reperfusion in some patients.

The activity of specific endogenous GAGs has only been characterized in a few cases and is mostly attributed to heparan sulfate in patients who have variceal bleeding, and probably during infection. In a single study, fluctuating levels of heparan and dermatan sulfate at all time points during transplant and up to 3 weeks after the operation were found in a pediatric cohort in all patients. Therefore, characterization of anticoagulant activity of specific GAGs needs to be explored in this group of patients. Prevention of infection remains essential to avoid worsening of coagulation in cirrhotics. However, specific pharmacologic treatment to reverse the HLE with protamine during liver transplant is still controversial, and the use of Neutralase, specific for cleaving endogenous heparinoids, used so far only during cardiac surgery, needs to be studied.

REFERENCES

1. Senzolo M, Burroughs AK. Hemostasis alterations in liver disease and liver transplantation. In: Kitchens G, Alving B, Kessler G, editors. Consultative hemostasis and thrombosis. Philadelphia: Saunders; 2007.
2. Senzolo M, Burra P, Cholongitas E, et al. New insights into the coagulopathy of liver disease and liver transplantation. World J Gastroenterol 2006;12(48): 7725–36.
3. Tripodi A, Salerno F, Chantarangkul V, et al. Evidence of normal thrombin generation in cirrhosis despite abnormal conventional coagulation tests. Hepatology 2005;41(3):553–8.
4. Tripodi A, Primignani M, Chantarangkul V, et al. Thrombin generation in patients with cirrhosis: the role of platelets. Hepatology 2006;44(2):440–5.
5. Bernard B, Grange JD, Khac EN, et al. Antibiotic prophylaxis for the prevention of bacterial infections in cirrhotic patients with gastrointestinal bleeding: a meta-analysis. Hepatology 1999;29(6):1655–61.
6. Goulis J, Patch D, Burroughs AK. Bacterial infection in the pathogenesis of variceal bleeding. Lancet 1999;353(9147):139–42.
7. Goulis J, Armonis A, Patch D, et al. Bacterial infection is independently associated with failure to control bleeding in cirrhotic patients with gastrointestinal hemorrhage. Hepatology 1998;27(5):1207–12.
8. Bernard B, Cadranel JF, Valla D, et al. Prognostic significance of bacterial infection in bleeding cirrhotic patients: a prospective study. Gastroenterology 1995; 108(6):1828–34.
9. Hou MC, Lin HC, Liu TT, et al. Antibiotic prophylaxis after endoscopic therapy prevents rebleeding in acute variceal hemorrhage: a randomized trial. Hepatology 2004;39(3):746–53.
10. Jun CH, Park CH, Lee WS, et al. Antibiotic prophylaxis using third generation cephalosporins can reduce the risk of early rebleeding in the first acute gastro-esophageal variceal hemorrhage: a prospective randomized study. J Korean Med Sci 2006;21(5):883–90.
11. Thalheimer U, Triantos CK, Samonakis DN, et al. Infection, coagulation, and variceal bleeding in cirrhosis. Gut 2005;54(4):556–63.
12. Grignani G, Maiolo A. Cytokines and hemostasis. Haematologica 2000;85(9): 967–72.
13. Violi F, Ferro D, Basili S, et al. Association between low-grade disseminated intravascular coagulation and endotoxemia in patients with liver cirrhosis. Gastroenterology 1995;109(2):531–9.
14. Plessier A, Denninger MH, Consigny Y, et al. Coagulation disorders in patients with cirrhosis and severe sepsis. Liver Int 2003;23(6):440–8.
15. Wong F, Bernardi M, Balk R, et al. Sepsis in cirrhosis: report on the 7th meeting of the International Ascites Club. Gut 2005;54(5):718–25.
16. Chau TN, Chan YW, Patch D, et al. Thrombelastographic changes and early rebleeding in cirrhotic patients with variceal bleeding. Gut 1998;43(2):267–71.

17. Papatheodoridis GV, Patch D, Webster GJ, et al. Infection and hemostasis in decompensated cirrhosis: a prospective study using thrombelastography. Hepatology 1999;29(4):1085–90.

18. Despotis GJ, Summerfield AL, Joist JH, et al. In vitro reversal of heparin effect with heparinase: evaluation with whole blood prothrombin time and activated partial thromboplastin time in cardiac surgical patients. Anesth Analg 1994;79(4): 670–4.

19. Tuman KJ, McCarthy RJ, Djuric M, et al. Evaluation of coagulation during cardiopulmonary bypass with a heparinase-modified thromboelastographic assay. J Cardiothorac Vasc Anesth 1994;8(2):144–9.

20. Montalto P, Vlachogiannakos J, Cox DJ, et al. Bacterial infection in cirrhosis impairs coagulation by a heparin effect: a prospective study. J Hepatol 2002; 37(4):463–70.

21. Zambruni A, Thalheimer U, Coppell J, et al. Endogenous heparin-like activity detected by anti-Xa assay in infected cirrhotic and non-cirrhotic patients. Scand J Gastroenterol 2004;39(9):830–6.

22. Guarner C, Soriano G, Tomas A, et al. Increased serum nitrite and nitrate levels in patients with cirrhosis: relationship to endotoxemia. Hepatology 1993;18(5): 1139–43.

23. Nielsen VG. Nitric oxide decreases coagulation protein function in rabbits as assessed by thromboelastography. Anesth Analg 2001;92(2):320–3.

24. Dhainaut JF, Marin N, Mignon A, et al. Hepatic response to sepsis: interaction between coagulation and inflammatory processes. Crit Care Med 2001;29(Suppl 7): S42–7.

25. Horne MK III, Stein CA, LaRocca RV, et al. Circulating glycosaminoglycan anticoagulants associated with suramin treatment. Blood 1988;71(2):273–9.

26. Murata K, Akashio K, Ochiai Y. Changes in acidic glycosaminoglycan components at different stages of human liver cirrhosis. Hepatogastroenterology 1984;31(6):261–5.

27. Weiss SJ. Tissue destruction by neutrophils. N Engl J Med 1989;320(6):365–76.

28. Cavari S, Vannucchi S. Glycosaminoglycans exposed on the endothelial cell surface. Binding of heparin-like molecules derived from serum. FEBS Lett 1993; 323(1–2):155–8.

29. Lamari FN, Militsopoulou M, Mitropoulou TN, et al. Analysis of glycosaminoglycan-derived disaccharides in biologic samples by capillary electrophoresis and protocol for sequencing glycosaminoglycans. Biomed Chromatogr 2002;16(2): 95–102.

30. Zmuda K, Neofotistos D, Ts'ao CH. Effects of unfractionated heparin, low-molecular-weight heparin, and heparinoid on thromboelastographic assay of blood coagulation. Am J Clin Pathol 2000;113(5):725–31.

31. Su H, Blain F, Musil RA, et al. Isolation and expression in Escherichia coli of hepB and hepC, genes coding for the glycosaminoglycan-degrading enzymes heparinase II and heparinase III, respectively, from Flavobacterium heparinum. Appl Environ Microbiol 1996;62(8):2723–34.

32. Yang VC, Linhardt RJ, Bernstein H, et al. Purification and characterization of heparinase from Flavobacterium heparinum. J Biol Chem 1985;260(3):1849–57.

33. Kang YG, Martin DJ, Marquez J, et al. Intraoperative changes in blood coagulation and thrombelastographic monitoring in liver transplantation. Anesth Analg 1985;64(9):888–96.

34. Kang Y. Thromboelastography in liver transplantation. Semin Thromb Hemost 1995;21(Suppl 4):34–44.

35. Bakker CM, Blankensteijn JD, Schlejen P, et al. The effects of long-term graft preservation on intraoperative hemostatic changes in liver transplantation. A comparison between orthotopic and heterotopic transplantation in the pig. HPB Surg 1994;7(4):265–80.

36. Bayly PJ, Thick M. Reversal of post-reperfusion coagulopathy by protamine sulphate in orthotopic liver transplantation. Br J Anaesth 1994;73(6):840–2.

37. Bellani KG, Estrin JA, Ascher NL, et al. Reperfusion coagulopathy during human liver transplantation. Transplant Proc 1987;19(4 Suppl 3):71–2.

38. Chapin JW, Peters KR, Winslow J, et al. Circulating heparin during liver transplantation. Transplant Proc 1993;25(2):1803.

39. Pivalizza EG, Abramson DC, King FS Jr. Thromboelastography with heparinase in orthotopic liver transplantation. J Cardiothorac Vasc Anesth 1998;12(3):305–8.

40. Kettner SC, Gonano C, Seebach F, et al. Endogenous heparin-like substances significantly impair coagulation in patients undergoing orthotopic liver transplantation. Anesth Analg 1998;86(4):691–5.

41. Auwerda JJ, Bac DJ, van't Veer MB, et al. Successful management of hemolysis in ABO-nonidentical orthotopic liver transplantation by steroid therapy: a case report. Transpl Int 1996;9(5):509–12.

42. Harding SA, Mallett SV, Peachey TD, et al. Use of heparinase modified thrombelastography in liver transplantation. Br J Anaesth 1997;78(2):175–9.

43. Agarwal S, Senzolo M, Melikian C, et al. The prevalence of a heparin-like effect shown on the thromboelastograph in patients undergoing liver transplantation. Liver Transpl 2008;14(6):855–60.

44. Senzolo M, Agarwal S, Zappoli P, et al. Heparin-like effect contributes to the coagulopathy in patients with acute liver failure undergoing liver transplatation. Liver Int 2008, in press.

45. McKee RF, Hodson S, Dawes J, et al. Plasma concentrations of endogenous heparinoids in portal hypertension. Gut 1992;33(11):1549–52.

46. Szende B, Lapis K, Kovalszky I, et al. Role of the modified (glycosaminoglycan producing) perisinusoidal fibroblasts in the CCl4-induced fibrosis of the rat liver. In Vivo 1992;6(4):355–61.

47. Colburn P, Buonassisi V. Anti-clotting activity of endothelial cell cultures and heparan sulfate proteoglycans. Biochem Biophys Res Commun 1982;104(1):220–7.

48. Bourin MC, Lindahl U. Glycosaminoglycans and the regulation of blood coagulation. Biochem J 1993;289(Pt 2):313–30.

49. Cavari S, Stramaccia L, Vannucchi S. Endogenous heparinase-sensitive anticoagulant activity in human plasma. Thromb Res 1992;67(2):157–65.

50. Trowbridge JM, Gallo RL. Dermatan sulfate: new functions from an old glycosaminoglycan. Glycobiology 2002;12(9):117R–25R.

51. Huntington JA. Mechanisms of glycosaminoglycan activation of the serpins in hemostasis. J Thromb Haemost 2003;1(7):1535–49.

52. Nader HB, Pinhal MA, Bau EC, et al. Development of new heparin-like compounds and other antithrombotic drugs and their interaction with vascular endothelial cells. Braz J Med Biol Res 2001;34(6):699–709.

53. Ofosu FA, Modi GJ, Smith LM, et al. Heparan sulfate and dermatan sulfate inhibit the generation of thrombin activity in plasma by complementary pathways. Blood 1984;64(3):742–7.

54. McGee M, Wagner WD. Chondroitin sulfate anticoagulant activity is linked to water transfer: relevance to proteoglycan structure in atherosclerosis. Arterioscler Thromb Vasc Biol 2003;23(10):1921–7.

55. Zancan P, Mourao PA. Venous and arterial thrombosis in rat models: dissociation of the antithrombotic effects of glycosaminoglycans. Blood Coagul Fibrinolysis 2004;15(1):45–54.

56. Senzolo M, Coppell J, Cholongitas E, et al. The effects of glycosaminoglycans on coagulation: a thromboelastographic study. Blood Coagul Fibrinolysis 2007; 18(3):227–36.

57. Senzolo M, Riddell A, Tuddenham E, et al. Endogenous heparinoids contribute to coagulopathy in patients with liver disease. J Hepatol 2008;48(2):371–2.

58. Khoory MS, Nesheim ME, Bowie EJ, et al. Circulating heparan sulfate proteoglycan anticoagulant from a patient with a plasma cell disorder. J Clin Invest 1980; 65(3):666–74.

59. Palmer RN, Rick ME, Rick PD, et al. Circulating heparan sulfate anticoagulant in a patient with a fatal bleeding disorder. N Engl J Med 1984;310(26):1696–9.

60. Wages DS, Staprans I, Hambleton J, et al. Structural characterization and functional effects of a circulating heparan sulfate in a patient with hepatocellular carcinoma. Am J Hematol 1998;58(4):285–92.

61. Tefferi A, Owen BA, Nichols WL, et al. Isolation of a heparin-like anticoagulant from the plasma of a patient with metastatic bladder carcinoma. Blood 1989; 74(1):252–4.

62. Ernst S, Langer R, Cooney CL, et al. Enzymatic degradation of glycosaminoglycans. Crit Rev Biochem Mol Biol 1995;30(5):387–444.

63. Senzolo M, Cholongitas E, Thalheimer U, et al. Heparinase I II and III modified thromboelastography for the detection of different glycosaminoglycans' effect in cirrhotics with bacterial infection. J Hepatol 2008;44(S2) [abstract].

64. Mitchell L, Superina R, Delorme M, et al. Circulating dermatan sulfate and heparan sulfate/heparin proteoglycans in children undergoing liver transplantation. Thromb Haemost 1995;74(3):859–63.

65. Ruiz-del-Arbol L, Urman J, Fernandez J, et al. Systemic, renal, and hepatic hemodynamic derangement in cirrhotic patients with spontaneous bacterial peritonitis. Hepatology 2003;38(5):1210–8.

66. Thalheimer U, Triantos C, Samonakis D, et al. Endogenous heparinoids in acute variceal bleeding. Gut 2005;54(2):310–1.

67. Stafford-Smith M, Lefrak EA, Qazi AG, et al. Efficacy and safety of heparinase I versus protamine in patients undergoing coronary artery bypass grafting with and without cardiopulmonary bypass. Anesthesiology 2005;103(2):229–40.

Tests of Coagulation in Liver Disease

Armando Tripodi, PhD

KEYWORDS

- Cirrhosis • Bleeding • Coagulation tests • Thrombin generation
- Fibrinolysis • Thromboelastography • Prothrombin time
- Activated partial thromboplastin time

Cirrhosis is characterized by a complex hemostatic defect including primary hemostasis, coagulation, and fibrinolysis.[1] This defect is considered responsible for the bleeding problems that often are associated with the disease, and the causal relationship between abnormal tests and bleeding has become an accepted paradigm. Accordingly, hepatologists order laboratory testing to assess the risk of bleeding and rely on the results to make decisions about the management of the coagulation disturbances, using procoagulant drugs as prophylactic or interventional measures (reviewed in Ref.[2]). Recent data, however, indicate that this presumed association might not be valid. This article reviews and appraises the clinical value of the main testing procedures related to coagulation, fibrinolysis, and thromboelastography.

COAGULATION

Cirrhosis is characterized by an impaired synthesis of all coagulation factors,[1] except for factor VIII[3] and von Willebrand's factor.[4] This defect usually is documented by the measurement of individual coagulation factors or by the prolongation of such global tests as the prothrombin time (PT) and the activated partial thromboplastin time (aPTT).

Prothrombin Time

The PT, also called "tissue factor–induced coagulation time," is a test developed by Armand Quick in 1935 for investigating patients with liver disease.[5] The test result consists of the time needed for the platelet-poor plasma to clot after the addition of tissue extracts (thromboplastin) and calcium chloride. The PT is responsive to congenital or acquired deficiencies of factors VII, X, V, and II and fibrinogen. The type of thromboplastin is the main determinant of the responsiveness of the test to the coagulation defect. Results can be expressed as simple coagulation times (in seconds) or as

Angelo Bianchi Bonomi Hemophilia and Thrombosis Center, Department of Internal Medicine, University Medical School and IRCCS Maggiore Hospital, Mangiagalli and Regina Elena Foundation, Via Pace 9, 20122 Milano, Italy
E-mail address: armando.tripodi@unimi.it

Clin Liver Dis 13 (2009) 55–61
doi:10.1016/j.cld.2008.09.002
1089-3261/08/$ – see front matter © 2009 Elsevier Inc. All rights reserved.

liver.theclinics.com

percentage activities interpolated from a dose–response curve constructed by testing increasing dilutions of a normal pooled plasma to which an arbitrary activity of 100% is assigned. Other ways of expressing results are the ratio (patient-to-normal coagulation time) and the international normalized ratio (INR), in which the ratio is raised to a power equal to the international sensitivity index (ISI) of the measuring system used for testing.

The INR is not a test but rather is a scale of values for the PT test that was introduced in 1983 as a means of harmonizing PT results across laboratories. The regular INR is expected to harmonize PT results only for patients taking vitamin K antagonists,[6] because the ISI needed to convert results usually is determined by means of plasma from patients taking vitamin K antagonists.[6] The use of the INR scale to harmonize results for patients who have liver disease requires appropriate determination of the relevant ISI value for this category of patients.[7,8]

Activated Partial Thromboplastin Time

The aPTT, developed in 1953[9] and modified in 1961,[10] is the time (in seconds) needed for the platelet-poor plasma to clot when mixed with a particulate or soluble activator of the contact coagulation factors (factor XII, pre-kallikrein, and high-molecular-weight kininogen) and negatively charged phospholipids as platelet substitutes. The aPTT is responsive to congenital or acquired deficiencies of all coagulation factors except factors VII and XIII. The type, concentration, and combination of activators and phospholipids determine the responsiveness of the test. The results, which usually are expressed as a coagulation time or a ratio (patient-to-normal coagulation time), vary according to the commercial measuring system used for testing; no standardization scheme has been devised to harmonize results across laboratories.

Clinical Value of Prothrombin Time and Activated Partial Thromboplastin Time in Cirrhosis

The PT and aPTT are used ostensibly to investigate patients who have cirrhosis even though these tests are known to be poor predictors of bleeding in this category of patients.[11–20] To explain this apparent paradox, it has been argued that the PT and aPTT might be inadequate to reflect the balance of coagulation as it occurs in vivo, especially in cirrhosis, a condition in which the levels of such naturally occurring anticoagulants as protein C and antithrombin are reduced in parallel with the procoagulants.[21] It also should be noted that protein C in vivo is activated by thrombin in cooperation with its endothelial receptor, thrombomodulin.[22] Plasma and reagents needed to perform PT and aPTT do not contain sufficient amounts of thrombomodulin. As a consequence, the activation of protein C is limited, and it cannot exert its full anticoagulant activity.[21] Therefore, it is reasonable to assume that PT and aPTT are responsive only to the thrombin generated as a function of procoagulants but are much less responsive to the inhibition of thrombin mediated by the anticoagulants. Accordingly, PT and aPTT should be regarded as suitable tests to investigate congenital deficiencies of procoagulants but not congenital deficiencies of anticoagulants or acquired deficiencies of both pro- and anticoagulants, as occurs in cirrhosis.[21] These reasons may be why the global coagulation tests are poor predictors of bleeding in patients who have cirrhosis. Indeed, the balance of pro- and anticoagulants in stable cirrhosis was found to be normal when assessed by thrombin generation measured in the presence of thrombomodulin,[21] and this balance was seen even though the PT and aPTT were prolonged.[21] Platelets contribute to the generation of thrombin;[23] therefore the occurrence of thrombocytopenia and/or thrombocytopathy often found in cirrhosis theoretically could affect the generation of thrombin in this condition. A recent study, however, showed that thrombin generation, when measured in platelet-rich plasma from stable cirrhotics in the presence of thrombomodulin, was indistinguishable from that of control subjects under the same experimental conditions, provided that the platelet levels were higher than 60 × 10⁹/L.[24]

The conclusion drawn from these studies is that coagulation in patients who have stable cirrhosis is normal if the platelet levels are sufficiently high to sustain the normal thrombin generation elicited by plasma. This conclusion might explain the poor efficacy shown by such antihemorrhagic agents as recombinant activated factor VII when used for patients who have chronic liver disease,[25–27] even though this agent shortens the PT. As a corollary, one may conclude that conventional coagulation tests are of little value for predicting bleeding in cirrhosis or for guiding decisions about the appropriate management of bleeding events in cirrhotic patients. If a test is needed at all in this condition, one of the leading candidates is thrombin generation assessed in the presence of thrombomodulin, provided there is sufficient fibrinogen.

Thrombin Generation Test

The thrombin generation test is a global test in which plasmatic coagulation is activated with small amounts of tissue factor as a trigger and phospholipids that act as platelet substitutes.[28,29] The thrombin generation curve (ie, the thrombin concentration versus time) (**Fig. 1**) is characterized by the lag phase, which occurs soon after the activation of coagulation, the peak of thrombin, the time to peak, and the area under the curve, which is called the "endogenous thrombin potential." The endogenous thrombin potential may be considered a measure of the amount of thrombin that a given plasma sample may generate under the specified experimental conditions and represents the balance between the pro- and anticoagulant proteins operating in plasma. The test mimics more closely than any other what occurs in vivo. It can be useful to assess the risk of bleeding in patients who have cirrhosis, but further clinical studies are needed to substantiate this hypothesis, especially for patients whose condition is complicated by bacterial infections or endothelial dysfunction. Until the results of such studies are available, clinicians responsible for patients who have cirrhosis should rely more heavily on their clinical judgment (history of previous bleeding,

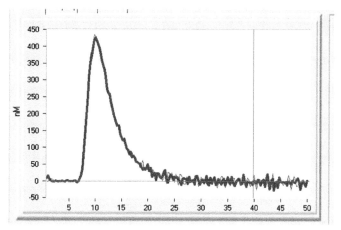

Fig. 1. Thrombin generation (nM thrombin versus time) curve. The area under the curve represents the endogenous thrombin potential.

hemodynamic alterations subsequent to portal hypertension, renal failure, and endothelial dysfunction) and less on the results of conventional global coagulation tests.

The Prothrombin Time as an Index of Prognosis in Cirrhosis

The PT also has been used over the years in combination with other clinical and laboratory parameters to calculate such prognostic indexes as the Child-Pugh[30] or the model of end-stage liver disease (MELD).[31] The MELD, in particular, has gained wide acceptance as an index of survival[31] and has been used to prioritize patients listed for liver transplantation.[32] The observations summarized in the previous paragraph on the unsuitability of the PT to predict bleeding do not subsume its usefulness in the prognosis of cirrhosis, which remains intact, provided results are expressed in the appropriate scale to ensure harmonization of results across laboratories.[33] More information on this topic is provided in the articles by Trotter and Kamath in this issue.

FIBRINOLYSIS

As shown in **Fig. 2**, fibrinolysis is a tightly regulated mechanism by which the proenzyme plasminogen is converted into the enzyme plasmin. The literature and textbooks state that cirrhosis is characterized by hyperfibrinolysis. This complex defect is documented at present by measuring the individual plasmatic components of fibrinolysis and, more rarely, through global tests. The measurement of the individual components cannot give a clear picture of the balance of fibrinolysis because of the complex interplay between activators and anti-activators that regulates the plasminogen–plasmin conversion. Reports in the literature show that cirrhotics may have increased levels of tissue plasminogen activator and its inhibitor but also can have decreased levels of plasminogen, antiplasmin, and factor XIII (reviewed in Ref.[2]).

Recent attention has focused on thrombin-activatable fibrinolysis inhibitor (TAFI), and researchers have speculated that its deficiency, a typical feature of cirrhosis, may explain the hyperfibrinolytic state often described in this condition. Recent investigations on this topic gave conflicting results, however. According to Lisman and colleagues,[34] deficiency of TAFI is not associated with increased plasma fibrinolysis, because the reduction of TAFI is counterbalanced by the concomitant decrease of the profibrinolytic factors. Conversely, according to Colucci and colleagues,[35] the deficiency of TAFI is associated with increased plasma fibrinolysis. A possible explanation for these conflicting findings may be the different designs of the global assays

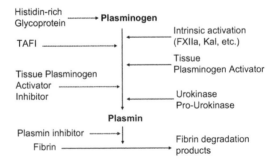

Fig. 2. Schematic representation of fibrinolysis. Solid and broken arrows represent profibrinolytic and antifibrinolytic factors, respectively. TAFI, thrombin activatable fibrinolysis inhibitor.

used by the two investigators to assess the balance of fibrinolysis. No commercial global assays for fibrinolysis are available, and standardization of homemade assays is difficult and beyond the expertise of the average clinical laboratory. In conclusion, these observations suggest that the measurement of individual components of the fibrinolytic pathway is unlikely to help; simple global tests representing the balance operating in vivo should be the developed and investigated in clinical trials to assess their value in predicting bleeding in patients who have cirrhosis.

THROMBOELASTOGRAPHY

Thromboelastography is a technique that can provide continuous observation and tracing of all the hemostatic functions that lead to clot formation and dissolution. It was developed many years ago as a means to investigate patients who had hemorrhagic disease and can be considered, at least in theory, as the prototype of a global test for hemostasis because it (allegedly) takes into account primary hemostasis, coagulation, and fibrinolysis. In the past, the use of this technique was limited somewhat by poor standardization, poor reproducibility, and the difficulty of interpreting the tracings and parameters.

Recently, the concepts of thromboelastography have been revisited and coupled with new computer technology. This combination, together with the design of new materials and equipment, has made modern thromboelastography more popular as a bedside tool, especially during such major surgical interventions as liver transplantation and cardiovascular procedures.[36] More recently, thromboelastography has been used to provide evidence for the generation of endogenous heparinoids as possible contributors to the coagulopathy in patients who have liver disease.[37] In this application thromboelastography using native blood could be useful in clinical practice to detect the anticoagulant effect of endogenous heparinoids and the associated hemorrhagic events. To be consistent with in vivo conditions, however, it should incorporate thrombomodulin to secure optimal protein C activation. Further work is urgently needed to explore the clinical application of this combined technology to optimize the use of potentially helpful therapeutics and to avoid unnecessary and potentially dangerous use of blood products and procoagulants.

SUMMARY

Although not yet entirely conclusive, all the observations presented here are consistent with the concept that the abnormality of coagulation in stable cirrhosis is more a myth than a reality. This understanding helps explain the apparent paradox of the prolonged global coagulation tests and their apparent poor prediction of bleeding in this setting and raises questions about the usefulness of conventional testing. Alternative tests mimicking more closely what occurs in vivo should be developed and investigated in appropriate clinical trials to determine their value in the management of bleeding in cirrhosis.

REFERENCES

1. Hedner U, Erhardtsen E. Hemostatic disorders in liver disease. In: Schiff ER, Sorrell MF, Maddrey WC, editors. Diseases of the liver. Philadelphia: Lippincott Williams and Wilkins; 2003. p. 625–35.
2. Caldwell SH, Hoffman M, Lisman T, et al. Coagulation disorders and hemostasis in liver disease: pathophysiology and critical assessment of current management. Hepatology 2006;44:1039–46.

3. Hollestelle MJ, Geertzen HG, Straatsburg IH, et al. Factor VIII expression in liver disease. Thromb Haemost 2004;91:267–75.
4. Lisman T, Bongers TN, Adelmeijer J, et al. Elevated levels of von Willebrand factor in cirrhosis support platelet adhesion despite reduced functional capacity. Hepatology 2006;44:53–61.
5. Quick AJ. The prothrombin in hemophilia and in obstructive jaundice. J Biol Chem 1935;109:73–4.
6. van den Besselaar AMHP, Poller L, Tripodi A. Guidelines for thromboplastins and plasmas used to control oral anticoagulant therapy (1999). WHO Tech Rep Ser 1999;889:64–93.
7. Tripodi A, Chantarangkul V, Primignani M, et al. The international normalized ratio calibrated for cirrhosis (INR$_{liver}$) normalizes prothrombin time results for model for end-stage liver disease calculation. Hepatology 2007;46:520–7.
8. Bellest L, Eschwege V, Poupon R, et al. A modified international normalized ratio as an effective way of prothrombin time standardization in hepatology. Hepatology 2007;46:528–34.
9. Langdell RD, Wagner RH, Brinkhous KM. Effect of antihemophilic factor on one-stage clotting tests; a presumptive test for hemophilia and a simple one-stage antihemophilic factor assay procedure. J Lab Clin Med 1953;41:637–47.
10. Proctor RR, Rapaport SI. The partial thromboplastin time with kaolin. A simple screening test for first stage plasma clotting factor deficiencies. Am J Clin Pathol 1961;36:212–9.
11. Schemmer P, Decker F, Dei-Anane G, et al. The vital threat of an upper gastrointestinal bleeding: risk factor analysis of 121 consecutive patients. World J Gastroenterol 2006;12:3597–601.
12. Ewe K. Bleeding after liver biopsy does not correlate with indices of peripheral coagulation. Dig Dis Sci 1981;26:388–93.
13. Dillon JF, Simpson KJ, Hayes PC. Liver biopsy bleeding time: an unpredictable event. J Gastroenterol Hepatol 1994;9:269–71.
14. Segal JB, Dzik WH. Paucity of studies to support that abnormal coagulation test results predict bleeding in the setting of invasive procedures: an evidence-based review. Transfusion 2005;45:1413–25.
15. Boks AL, Brommer EJ, Schalm SW, et al. Hemostasis and fibrinolysis in severe liver failure and their relation to hemorrhage. Hepatology 1986;6:79–86.
16. Diaz LK, Teruya J. Liver biopsy. N Engl J Med 2001;344:2030.
17. Grabau CM, Crago SF, Hoff LK, et al. Performance standards for therapeutic abdominal paracentesis. Hepatology 2004;40:484–8.
18. Terjung B, Lemnitzer I, Dumoulin FL, et al. Bleeding complications after percutaneous liver biopsy. An analysis of risk factors. Digestion 2003;67:138–45.
19. McGill DB, Rakela J, Zinsmeister AR, et al. A 21 year experience with major hemorrhage after percutaneous liver biopsy. Gastroenterology 1990;99:1396–400.
20. Bravo AA, Sheth SG, Chopra S. Liver biopsy. N Engl J Med 2001;344:495–500.
21. Tripodi A, Salerno F, Chantarangkul V, et al. Evidence of normal thrombin generation in cirrhosis despite abnormal conventional coagulation tests. Hepatology 2005;41:553–8.
22. Dahlback B. Progress in the understanding of the protein C anticoagulant pathway. Int J Hematol 2004;79:109–16.
23. Bevers EM, Comfurius P, Zwaal RF. Platelet procoagulant activity: physiological significance and mechanisms of exposure. Blood Rev 1991;5:146–54.
24. Tripodi A, Primignani M, Chantarangkul V, et al. Thrombin generation in patients with cirrhosis: the role of platelets. Hepatology 2006;44:440–5.

25. Bosch J, Thabut D, Bendtsen F, et al. Recombinant factor VIIa for upper gastro-intestinal bleeding in patients with cirrhosis: a randomized, double-blind trial. Gastroenterology 2004;127:1123–30.
26. Lodge JP, Jonas S, Jones RM, et al. Efficacy and safety of repeated perioperative doses of recombinant factor VIIa in liver transplantation. Liver Transpl 2005;11:973–9.
27. Planinsic RM, van der Meer J, Testa G, et al. Safety and efficacy of a single bolus administration of recombinant factor VIIa in liver transplantation due to chronic liver disease. Liver Transpl 2005;11:895–900.
28. Hemker HC, Giesen P, Al Dieri R, et al. Calibrated automated thrombin generation measurement in clotting plasma. Pathophysiol Haemost Thromb 2003;33:4–15.
29. Chantarangkul V, Clerici M, Bressi A, et al. Thrombin generation assessed as en-dogenous thrombin potential (ETP) in patients with hypo- or hyper-coagulability. Effects of phospholipids, tissue factor and residual platelets on the measurement performed in platelet-poor and platelet-rich plasma. Haematologica 2003;88:547–54.
30. Pugh RN, Murray-Lyon IM, Dawson JL, et al. Transection of the oesophagus for bleeding oesophageal varices. Br J Surg 1973;60:646–9.
31. Malinchoc M, Kamath PS, Gordon FD, et al. A model to predict poor survival in patients undergoing transjugular intrahepatic portosystemic shunts. Hepatology 2000;31:864–71.
32. Wiesner R, Edwards E, Freeman R, et al. United Network for Organ Sharing Liver Disease Severity Score Committee. Model for end-stage liver disease (MELD) and allocation of donor liver. Gastroenterology 2003;124:91–6.
33. Tripodi A, Chantarangkul V, Mannucci PM. The international normalized ratio to prioritize patients for liver transplantation. Problems and possible solutions. J Thromb Haemost In press.
34. Lisman T, Leebeek FW, Mosnier LO, et al. Thrombin-activatable fibrinolysis inhib-itor deficiency in cirrhosis is not associated with increased plasma fibrinolysis. Gastroenterology 2001;121:131–9.
35. Colucci M, Binetti BM, Branca MG, et al. Deficiency of thrombin activatable fibrinolysis inhibitor in cirrhosis is associated with increased plasma fibrinolysis. Hepatology 2003;38:230–7.
36. Koh MB, Hunt BJ. The management of perioperative bleeding. Blood Rev 2003;17:179–85.
37. Montalto P, Vlachogiannakos J, Cox DJ, et al. Bacterial infections in cirrhosis impairs coagulation by a heparin effect: a prospective study. J Hepatol 2002;37:463–7.

The International Normalized Ratio of Prothrombin Time in the Model for End-Stage Liver Disease Score: A Reliable Measure

Patrick S. Kamath, MD*, W. Ray Kim, MD

KEYWORDS

- Cirrhosis • Liver transplantation • Prognostic models
- Portal hypertension • Survival

The Model for End-stage Liver Disease (MELD), created from a cohort of patients undergoing transjugular intrahepatic portosystemic shunts,[1] has been demonstrated to be an excellent predictor of survival in patients who have end-stage liver disease.[2,3] The MELD score is derived from the international normalized ratio (INR) of prothrombin time, serum creatinine, and serum total bilirubin using the following formula:

$$MELD = 9.57 \times \ln(cr) + 3.78 \times \ln(bili) + 11.20 \times \ln(INR) + 6.43$$

The major use of the MELD score in the United States, and also worldwide, is to prioritize the allocation of organs for liver transplant among patients who have chronic liver disease, because of the proven ability of the MELD system to rank patients according to risk for 3-month mortality. Of the three variables in the MELD score, the INR carries the most weight. Therefore, it is important that the INR be measured reliably. An inappropriate determination of the INR would result in an incorrect MELD score, thereby putting some patients listed for liver transplant at a disadvantage.

To understand the pitfalls in the determination of the INR, it is necessary to know the basis on which the INR system was created. The INR is a way of mathematically transforming the prothrombin time in seconds to a ratio. It was hoped that this system would eliminate the variation among laboratories in expressing the prothrombin time, because

Miles and Shirley Fiterman Center for Digestive Diseases, Mayo Clinic, College of Medicine, 200 First Street SW, Rochester, MN 55905, USA
* Corresponding author.
E-mail address: kamath.patrick@mayo.edu (P.S. Kamath).

Clin Liver Dis 13 (2009) 63–66
doi:10.1016/j.cld.2008.09.001
1089-3261/08/$ – see front matter © 2009 Elsevier Inc. All rights reserved.

patients on anticoagulation often obtained different readings from different laborato-ries. The INR for prothrombin time is derived by dividing the patient's prothrombin time by a control mean normal prothrombin time (MNPT), and the product is raised to the international sensitivity index (ISI) for thromboplastin. The ISI is provided by the manufacturer and varies between 1 and 3 worldwide, with most thromboplastins cur-rently available in the United States having an ISI closer to 1.

The INR system has been validated in patients on stable anticoagulation.[4] The INR, however, has also been used in place of the prothrombin time to determine severity of liver disease, even though a significant difference exists between the abnormalities in coagulation factors in patients who have liver disease and those in patients on warfa-rin. In liver disease, a deficiency may exist in fibrinogen, prothrombin (factor II), and factors V, VII, IX, and X, and components of the anticoagulant system, such as protein C and protein S. On the other hand, patients on warfarin have a decrease only in the vitamin K–derived factors, namely factors II, VII, IX, and X. Thus, patients who have liver disease have a significantly more complex coagulopathy than patients on warfa-rin because they have, in addition, a defect in anticoagulant factors, factor V, and pos-sibly fibrinogen synthesis. The INR may vary in liver disease because of causes that are generic and causes specific to liver disease.[5,6]

GENERIC CAUSES OF VARIATION IN THE INTERNATIONAL NORMALIZED RATIO

Generic causes of variation in the INR are related to incorrect determination of the MNPT, using an arithmetic mean rather than a geometric mean. Differences may also exist between the sodium citrate concentration used to determine the ISI by the manufacturer and the sodium citrate concentration used in the local laboratory. The ISI is typically calibrated for each reagent/instrument combination. Because dif-ferent instruments use different end points (manual, photo-optical, or mechanical methods), an incorrect instrument/reagent combination will also give an erroneous ISI.[7] The international reference preparation for calibration of instruments may also be chosen incorrectly, demonstrated by laboratories noting an incorrect calibration of the commercial agent against the international reference preparation.

The ISI is a major determinant of the INR. Each manufacturer determines the ISI of the thromboplastin in reference to a World Health Organization reference thrombo-plastin. More than 25 different commercially available thromboplastins need to be cali-brated locally. If the INR results on certified plasmas produce an INR that is different from the certified plasma INR by greater than 15%, the local-system ISI should not be adopted. Moreover, the coefficient of variation between determinations should be 3% or less, and if it exceeds 3%, the locally calibrated ISI cannot be considered valid. These important details are sometimes overlooked in laboratories, which results in an incorrect INR determination.

LIVER-SPECIFIC CAUSES OF VARIATION IN THE INTERNATIONAL NORMALIZED RATIO

The liver-specific causes of an incorrect INR are related to the fact that the ISI has been standardized for patients on warfarin therapy (see also the article by Tripodi in this issue). Because patients who have liver disease have more complex coagulop-athy, the ISI as calibrated for warfarin therapy may not be applicable to liver disease.

THE MODEL FOR END-STAGE LIVER DISEASE AS A PREDICTOR OF SURVIVAL

On the other hand, virtually every study that has looked at the MELD score as a predic-tor of survival has demonstrated that the MELD score, using the INR with ISI calibrated for patients on warfarin, has a 'c' statistic of approximately 0.8, indicating excellent discrimination. Although the current method of measuring INR has drawbacks, the INR is the only standardized method currently available in the United States for expressing the prothrombin time. Therefore, the INR, a reliable measure of prothrombin time in patients on anticoagulation, will also continue to be a means of expressing severity of liver disease.

The ISI is assigned to each batch of thromboplastin based on the prothrombin time in patients on warfarin anticoagulation. The ISI has not previously been calibrated based on prolongation of prothrombin time in patients who have chronic liver disease. Two recent studies have demonstrated that if thromboplastins are calibrated using plasma from patients who have cirrhosis (rather than plasma from patients on warfarin), the variability in measurement of the INR is largely eliminated.[8–10] The MELD scores using the INR obtained with recalibrated ISI were more reproducible in the patients who had cirrhosis who were studied.

A change to a laboratory system that uses an ISI calibrated to patients who have liver disease is likely to eliminate, to a great extent, the variation from laboratory to laboratory currently noted in the INR. Therefore, significant changes need to be made in the laboratory community to have two different prothrombin times, one for patients on oral anticoagulation and the other for patients who have liver disease ($INR_{vitamin K}$ antagonists and INR_{liver}).

SUMMARY

Currently, the ISI used in clinical laboratories to calculate the INR is not calibrated based on prolongation of prothrombin time in patients who have chronic liver disease. As a result, variation in the conventionally measured INR (using warfarin-derived standards to determine the thromboplastin ISI) has been well documented in patients who have liver disease. Despite this limitation, virtually every study that has looked at the MELD score as a predictor of survival has demonstrated that the MELD score using the conventional INR possesses excellent survival discrimination. This fact, along with the wide availability of this simple test, provides a strong argument for its continued use in survival estimations and thus organ allocation in advanced liver disease. Indeed, experts have recommended that the INR should not be removed from the MELD but rather, should be recalculated in patients who have chronic liver disease. If the ISI is calculated from standards based on chronic liver disease to provide the INR_{liver}, it is likely to provide an even more accurate measurement. It is anticipated that in the future, the variations in the prothrombin time and, therefore, the MELD score from laboratory to laboratory, will be greatly reduced by incorporation of this technique. Meanwhile, the current MELD calculation, using a conventionally determined INR, remains a proved, valid, and clinically useful tool in predicting survival in end-stage liver disease.

REFERENCES

1. Malinchoc M, Kamath PS, Gordon F, et al. A model to predict poor survival in patients undergoing transjugular intrahepatic portosystemic shunts. Hepatology 2000;31:864–71.
2. Kamath PS, Wiesner R, Malinchoc M, et al. A model to predict survival in patients with end-stage liver disease. Hepatology 2001;33:464–70.
3. Wiesner R, Edwards E, Freeman R, et al. United Network for Organ Sharing Liver Disease Severity Score Committee. Model for end-stage liver disease (MELD) and allocation of donor livers. Gastroenterology 2003;124:91–6.

4. Kirkwood T. Calibration of reference thromboplastins and standardization of the prothrombin time ratio. Thromb Haemost 1983;49:238–44.
5. van den Besselaar A, Barrowcliffe T, Houbouyan-Reveillard L, et al. Subcommittee on control of anticoagulation of the scientific and standardization committee of the ISTH. Guidelines on preparation, certification, and use of certified plasmas for ISI calibration and INR determination. J Thromb Haemost 2004;2:1946–53.
6. Trotter J, Brimhall B, Arjal R, et al. Specific laboratory methodologies achieve higher model for endstage liver disease (MELD) scores for patients listed for liver transplantation. Liver Transplantation 2004;10:995–1000.
7. Anonymous. Procedures for validation of INR and local calibration of PT/INR systems: approved guideline. Clinical and Laboratory Standards Institute 2004; 25:23.
8. Bellest L, Eschwege V, Poupon R, et al. A modified international normalized ratio as an effective way of prothrombin time standardization in hepatology. Hepatology 2007;46:528–34.
9. Tripodi A, Chantarangkul V, Primignani M, et al. International normalized ratio calibrated for cirrhosis (INR liver) normalizes prothrombin time results for model for end-stage liver disease calculation. Hepatology 2007;46:520–7.
10. Marlar RA. Determining the model for end-stage liver disease with better accuracy: neutralizing the international normalized ratio pitfalls. Hepatology 2007;46:295–6.

International Normalized Ratio of Prothrombin Time in the Model for End-stage Liver Disease Score: An Unreliable Measure

Russ Arjal, MD, James F. Trotter, MD*

KEYWORDS

• Liver transplant • Allocation • MELD • Outcomes • INR

The current basis for deceased donor (DD) liver allocation is the Model for End-stage Liver Disease (MELD) score, which is an objective means of predicting 90-day patient survival. The MELD score was originally designed to predict short-term survival after transjugular intrahepatic portosystemic shunt.[1] At the same time that the MELD score was developed, a rancorous debate emerged, based on the perceived lack of equity in nationwide liver allocation. The Institute of Medicine (IOM)[2] undertook a comprehensive review of liver allocation and made the following broad conclusions regarding liver transplantation:

1. Organs should be allocated to candidates with the greatest medical need.
2. Waiting time is irrelevant to transplant need and should be removed as a determinant.
3. An objective means of prioritizing candidates should be developed and used.
4. National parity for organ allocation is a desired goal.

The MELD score met the criteria set forth by the IOM in that it identified patients with the highest risk for short-term mortality (greatest need), lacked waiting time as a determinant, and ostensibly included only objective laboratory determinants. Compared with the previous means of liver allocation, the MELD score proved to be far superior

---

Division of Gastroenterology/Hepatology, University of Colorado Health Sciences Center, 1635 N. Ursula, B-154, Aurora, CO 80045, USA
* Corresponding author.
E-mail address: james.trotter@uchsc.edu (J.F. Trotter).

Clin Liver Dis 13 (2009) 67–71
doi:10.1016/j.cld.2008.09.009
1089-3261/08/$ – see front matter © 2009 Elsevier Inc. All rights reserved.

and was therefore adopted by the United Network for Organ Sharing as a means of prioritizing candidates for DD liver transplant in February 2002.[3–5]

MODEL FOR END-STAGE LIVER DISEASE DETERMINANTS

A stated advantage of the MELD score is that it is derived from "generalizable, verifiable, and easily obtained variables," namely, total bilirubin, creatinine, and international normalized ratio (INR)*.[3] In addition, one of the apparent advantages of organ allocation using the MELD score is the absence of subjective determinants, which were included in the Child-Turcotte-Pugh (CTP) score (severity of encephalopathy and ascites).[6] As a result, organ allocation is more equitable and purportedly, no means exists to use subjective criteria to increase priority for transplant, a problem that plagued the pre-MELD organ allocation scheme.

However, evidence indicates that the determinants that constitute the MELD score may not be as objective as originally reported. Specifically, serum creatinine may be altered by serum bilirubin values.[7] That is, patients who have severe jaundice may have different serum creatinine levels (and therefore a variable MELD score and prioritization for transplant) based on the selection of the laboratory methodology used in the creatinine assay. In addition, compared with men, women with the same level of renal dysfunction have lower serum creatinine values and therefore lower MELD scores and a lower transplant priority.[8] Finally, the INR, which has the highest multiplicative factor of the three MELD determinants, is significantly altered based simply on the selection of laboratory methodology.[9,10]

LIMITATIONS OF THE INTERNATIONAL NORMALIZED RATIO

The INR was never designed or intended for its current role in the MELD score. In fact, as discussed below, the test characteristics of the INR are poorly suited for its inclusion as a determinant in the MELD score. The INR was originally devised to standardize anticoagulation therapy after hematologists noted large and clinically relevant interlaboratory variations in prothrombin time in their anticoagulated patients. These variations led to difficulties in adjusting coumadin doses when patients had prothrombin times measured at different locations, and in standardizing the degree of anticoagulation in patients across the country. Most of the variation in prothrombin time is due to the variable sensitivity of thromboplastin reagents used in its determination. Therefore, the INR was developed to normalize the variable sensitivities of thromboplastin and is intended to return a value as if the prothrombin time were assayed using the standard World Health Organization thromboplastin regent. The INR is defined as (patient prothrombin time/control prothrombin time)^{ISI}, where ISI is international sensitivity index and control prothrombin values are generated from patients who received coumadin therapy.[11,12] Although theoretically normalizing the variable sensitivity in thromboplastin reagents, the INR provides an imperfect correction. That is, according to the College of American Pathologists' quality-control tests in coumadinzed patients, standardized specimens have a coefficient of variation of 13% INR values for laboratories that participated in proficiency testing.[13]

---

*MELD score = 10 (0.957 ln (Cr,mg/dL) + 0.378 ln (bilirubin, mg/dL) + 1.12 ln (INR) + 0.643), where laboratory values less than 1.0 are set to 1.0 for purposes of the MELD score calculation and the maximum serum creatinine considered within the MELD score equation is 4.0 mg/dL.

THE INTERNATIONAL NORMALIZED RATIO IN LIVER DISEASE

In liver patients, the variation in INR values among different assays is even greater. Kovacs and colleagues[14] measured mean INR using three different thromboplastin reagents in 28 patients who had liver impairment compared with patients receiving coumadin. Although significant difference existed between the mean INR values in the control patients, the liver patients demonstrated a 29% difference in mean INR ($P = .0001$). Denson and colleagues[15] reported similar results comparing three thromboplastin reagents in 20 liver patients, finding a 25% difference in mean INR. Robert and Chazouillères[16] measured INR using seven different thromboplastins in 27 patients who had liver failure and 29 patients on oral anticoagulants. Although no difference existed in mean INR for patients on anticoagulants, they noted a 78% difference in mean INR (ranging from 2.3 to 4.1) for the liver patients ($P = .007$). The difference was most pronounced with higher INR values, with an upper range varying from 5.2 to 14.3 between reagents.

These large variations in INR (and therefore MELD score) would occur in the patients with the highest MELD scores and the highest priority for transplant. The authors evaluated variations in INR and MELD scores in 29 patients listed for liver transplant using three different laboratory methodologies for measuring INR. A significant 26% difference occurred in INR, and a 21% difference in corresponding MELD score ($P<.05$).[9] In a larger follow-up study, they measured variation in five "standard" INR samples at 14 representative clinical laboratories across the United States. They found a wide range in INR values in each of the "standard" samples that corresponded to differences in MELD score up to 9 points.[10]

THE "INTERNATIONAL NORMALIZED RATIO PROBLEM"

With a growing recognition of "the INR problem" as it relates to the MELD score, investigators have begun to suggest remedies. Two recent studies have demonstrated that the large interlaboratory variation associated with INR values in liver patients may be resolved by using a different calibration technique for ISI.[17,18] Clinical laboratories routinely calibrate an ISI for each thromboplastin reagent against a reference preparation. Typically, the ISI is derived from the regression line of the logarithm of prothrombin time of the test reagent plotted against the logarithm of prothrombin time of the reference reagent across a wide range of values using specimens from normal and anticoagulated patients. Tripodi and colleagues[17] demonstrated the important difference of calibrating the ISI using specimens from liver patients, as compared with anticoagulated patients (ie, those receiving a vitamin K antagonist (VKA) such as coumadin). These investigators calculated an ISI(liver) by substituting in the calibration the plasmas from VKA patients with plasmas from patients who had cirrhosis. The mean INR(VKA) obtained with seven thromboplastins was significantly different ($P<.001$). However, the mean INR using ISI(liver) showed no difference. The investigators concluded that this alternative thromboplastin calibration technique (using plasmas from patients who have cirrhosis instead of from VKA patients) may resolve the problem of INR variability in patients who have liver disease.

However, implementing this "repair" may have substantial problems because clinical laboratories would have to (1) prepare a separate INR formula for liver patients and (2) prospectively identify these samples for a separate INR determination in liver transplant candidates.[19] This process would be particularly difficult in clinical laboratories outside the transplant centers, where 50% of transplant candidates have their blood analyzed[10] and where measuring INR for MELD score calculation would likely represent a tiny fraction of their overall business activity.

Another means of addressing the "INR problem" would be simply to remove it as a determinant from the MELD score altogether. Evidence indicates that INR could be removed from the MELD score without a significant reduction in its ability to predict 90-day mortality. Heuman and colleagues[20] reported that the c-statistic for MELD-XI (without INR) for 90-day mortality (0.83) was not significantly different than for MELD (0.84). The investigators concluded that the MELD-XI is nearly as accurate as MELD and should be used in anticoagulated patients listed for transplant.

PERSPECTIVE

When the MELD score was developed, its originators made a careful comparison of the test characteristics between determinants in the CTP score (the basis of the system of DD liver allocation before MELD) and MELD score. In fact, they recognized the importance of interlaboratory variation and how this variation could adversely alter assessment of patients: "The normal range of albumin across the Unites States varies from 2.9 to 4.5 g/dL in some laboratories to 3.8 to 5.1 g/dL at other laboratories. Because of this variability, a patient with a 5% decrease in albumin synthesis will be given 1 point in the CTP system in a laboratory where the lower limit of normal for albumin is 3.8 g/dL (5% decrease = albumin 3.6/dL), but 3 points if the albumin is measured in a laboratory where the lower limit of normal is 2.9 g/dL (5% decrease = albumin 2.8 g/dL)."[3]

Although the MELD "mavens" clearly recognized the importance of interlaboratory variation in albumin vis-à-vis assessment of disease severity, it is unclear whether it was fully appreciated in the case of the INR. Based on its presumed "standardization," the INR was held forth as a better test than the prothrombin time. The investigators noted that prothrombin time varied significantly among clinical laboratories: "The prothrombin time in seconds, which is used in the CTP classification, however, depends on the sensitivity of the thromboplastin reagent used (International Sensitivity Index, ISI) and, based on this sensitivity, the prothrombin time in seconds can vary greatly from laboratory to laboratory."[3] However, it is not clear if they fully appreciated the wide interlaboratory variation in the INR. They noted that "the prothrombin time is currently standardized and reported in most places worldwide as the INR for prothrombin time" and that the INR is "standardized across the country."[3]

SUMMARY

Liver allocation under the MELD system is a vast improvement over the prior allocation scheme. However, published studies have refuted the United Network for Organ Sharing statement that "the MELD and PELD [Pediatric End-stage Liver Disease] formulas are simple, objective and verifiable and yield consistent results whenever the score is calculated."[21] In particular, wide inter-laboratory variation exists in the most heavily weighted MELD determinant, the INR. Whether this variation impacts the equitable distribution of DD livers is unclear. However, this variation has the potential to detract from the expressed purpose of MELD-based allocation, which is to prioritize liver transplant candidates across the country with parity using an objective scoring system. As a result, this issue deserves a formal analysis to measure its impact on organ allocation. "Basing organ allocation on a system that has been derived from a much more evidence-based approach, however, will make it possible to scrutinize more rigorously the results of the system and more precisely apply appropriate changes."[4]

REFERENCES

1. Malinchoc M, Kamath PS, Gordon FD, et al. A model to predict poor survival in patients undergoing transjugular intrahepatic portosystemic shunts. Hepatology 2000;31:864–71.
2. Institute of Medicine Committee on Organ Procurement and Policy. Organ procurement and transplantation: assessing current policies and the potential impact of the DHHS final rule. Washington, DC: National Academy Press; 1999:1–29.
3. Kamath PS, Wiesner RH, Malinchoc M, et al. A model to predict survival in patients with end-stage liver disease. Hepatology 2001;33:464–70.
4. Wiesner R, Edwards E, Freeman R, et al. Model for end-stage liver disease (MELD) and allocation of donor liver. Gastroenterology 2003;124:91–6.
5. Freeman RB, Wiesner R, Harper A, et al. The new allocation system: moving toward evidence-based transplantation policy. Liver Transpl 2002;8:851–8.
6. Kamath PS, Kim WR. The model for end-stage liver disease (MELD). Hepatology 2007;45:797–805.
7. Cholongitas E, Marelli L, Kerry A, et al. Different methods of creatinine measurement significantly affect MELD scores. Liver Transpl 2007;13:523–9.
8. Cholongitas E, Marelli L, Kerry A, et al. Female liver transplant recipients with the same GFR as male recipients have lower MELD scores-a systematic bias. Am J Transplant 2007;7:685–92.
9. Trotter JF, Brimhall B, Arjal R, et al. Specific laboratory methodologies achieve higher model for end-stage liver disease (MELD) scores for patients listed for liver transplantation. Liver Transpl 2004;10:995–1000.
10. Trotter JF, Olson J, Lefkowitz J, et al. Changes in international normalized ratio (INR) and model for endstage liver disease (MELD) based on selection of clinical laboratory. Am J Transplant 2007;7:1624–8.
11. Hirsh J, Poller L. The international normalized ratio. Arch Intern Med 1994;154:282–8.
12. Kirkwood TB. Calibration of reference thromboplastins and standardization of the prothrombin time ratio. Thromb Haemost 1983;49:238–44.
13. Olson JD, Brandt JT, Chandler WL, et al. Laboratory reporting for the international normalized ratio: progress and problems. Arch Pathol Lab Med 2007;131:1641–7.
14. Kovacs MH, Wong A, MacKinnon K, et al. Assessment of the validity of the INR system for patients with liver impairment. Thromb Haemost 1994;71:727–30.
15. Denson KWE, Reed SV, Haddon ME, et al. Comparative studies of rabbit and human recombinant tissue factor reagents. Thromb Res 1999;94:255–61.
16. Robert A, Chazouilleres O. Prothrombin time in liver failure: time, ratio, activity percentage, or international normalized ratio. Hepatology 1996;24:1392–4.
17. Tripodi A, Chantarangkul V, Primignani M, et al. The international normalized ratio calibrated for cirrhosis (INR_{liver}) normalizes prothrombin time results for model for end-stage liver disease calculation. Hepatology 2007;46:528–34.
18. Bellest L, Eschwege V, Poupon R, et al. A modified international normalized ratio of prothrombin time standardization in hepatology. Hepatology 2007;46:520–7.
19. Marlar R. Determining the model for end-stage liver disease with better accuracy: neutralizing the international normalized ratio pitfalls. Hepatology 2007;46:295–6.
20. Heuman DM, Mihas AA, Habib A, et al. MELD-XI: a rational approach to "sickest first" liver transplantation in cirrhotic patients requiring anticoagulant therapy. Liver Transpl 2007;13:30–7.
21. United Network for Organ Sharing. Available at: http://www.unos.org/Shared ContentDocumens/Revised_MELDPELD_2003(2).pdf. Accessed December 20, 2005.

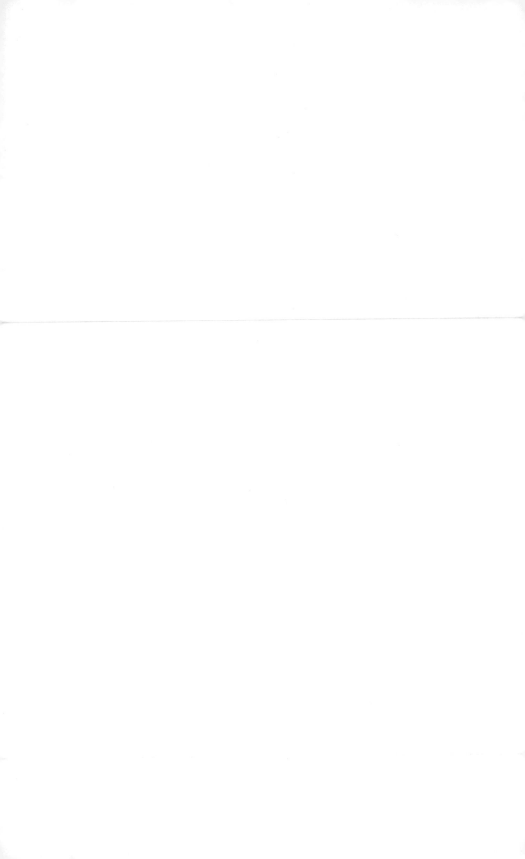

Blood Products, Volume Control, and Renal Support in the Coagulopathy of Liver Disease

Curtis K. Argo, MD, MS[a],*, Rasheed A. Balogun, MD[b]

KEYWORDS
- Blood products • Plasma • Transfusion
- Renal replacement therapy • Volume contraction

Management of coagulopathy in patients who have liver disease remains challenging, and recent studies cast serious doubt on the use of the international normalized ratio (INR) as a reliable indicator of bleeding risk, and thus it is also questionable as a target for meaningful prophylactic intervention. This development has raised further questions concerning past tenets of the use of plasma and blood transfusion before procedures or with acute hemorrhage. This article discusses the use of blood products, namely plasma, in patients who have cirrhosis and the overlap with volume control and renal failure. Although this view of plasma use is critical overall, the authors realize that specific situations exist when replacement therapy is warranted, particularly when fibrinogen levels are low. More research is needed, however, to better use factor replacement particularly newer procoagulant agents (see article by Shah and colleagues elsewhere in this issue), develop better targets of therapy in light of the limitations of the INR (see article by Tripodi elsewhere in this issue), and identify the potential complications of plasma and blood transfusion. The novel concepts of volume contraction and blood conservation therapies are also addressed.

PLASMA TRANSFUSION AS TREATMENT OF COAGULOPATHY

Use of plasma-based blood products has been a dogmatic treatment of the coagulopathy of liver disease. Randomized clinical trials provide little support, however, for

---

[a] University of Virginia, Department of Medicine, Division of Gastroenterology and Hepatology, Box 800708, Charlottesville, VA, USA
[b] University of Virginia, Department of Medicine, Division of Nephrology, Charlottesville, VA, USA
* Corresponding author.
E-mail address: cka3d@virginia.edu (C.K. Argo).

Clin Liver Dis 13 (2009) 73–85
doi:10.1016/j.cld.2008.09.007
1089-3261/08/$ – see front matter © 2009 Elsevier Inc. All rights reserved.

using plasma before invasive procedures, except when a bleeding diathesis is clearly indicated.[1] Three main products are predominant in this therapeutic setting: fresh frozen plasma (FFP) (frozen within 8 hours of collection), plasma frozen within 24 hours (FP24), and thawed plasma (refrigerated >24 hours after thawing and possibly used for up to 5 days). These different preparations vary slightly in factor levels.

Supply needs, especially with the shift to male-only donors to decrease transfusion-related acute lung injury (TRALI), have caused most suppliers to shift to FP24. Although plasma is commonly used in patients who have cirrhosis with prolonged INR, injudicious use should be regarded as a risk and liability in light of the limitations of the INR and the risks associated with plasma use.[2] Moreover, the amount of FFP requested is typically inadequate to replace deficient clotting factors in most patients who have cirrhosis.[3] For example, four units of plasma with a volume of roughly 1 L increases most clotting factors by only approximately 10%, leaving typical patients who have coagulopathic cirrhosis with a level of factors still in the range associated with INR prolongation.

An alternative to plasma products includes cryoprecipitate, which is especially useful if the fibrinogen level is depressed (<100–120 mg/dL) and when volume control is problematic. However, as with newer agents such as prothrombin complex concentrates, more investigation is needed to determine how best to use these alternative therapies.

TRANSFUSION-RELATED LUNG INJURY

TRALI is most frequently linked to FFP and platelet transfusion because of high concentrations of antileukocyte alloantibodies compared with other blood products.[4] Consensus criteria for TRALI include onset within 6 hours of the transfusion, acute-onset hypoxemia, bilateral infiltrates, normal or low central venous pressure, and no underlying previous lung injury (**Fig. 1**).[5] TRALI has a 5% to 10% mortality rate and occurs up to 12 times more commonly with FFP transfusion than other blood products.[6,7]

One single-center prospective cohort study showed that a preexisting clinical history of alcohol abuse and liver disease conferred higher risk for TRALI.[8] Although recipient-related factors have not received much additional attention in the literature, TRALI is widely perceived to be underreported in this severely ill population in whom

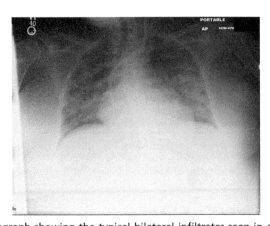

Fig. 1. Chest radiograph showing the typical bilateral infiltrates seen in a patient who has TRALI. This patient had undergone packed red cell transfusion 4 hours before this radiograph, when she abruptly developed increased oxygen requirements.

pulmonary edema may be multifactorial and is often attributed to fluid overload by default. TRALI accounts for approximately half of transfusion-associated acute respiratory failure in critical care patients. Transfusion-associated circulatory overload (TACO), which more often complicates packed red cell transfusion, accounts for the other half (**Table 1**).[9,10]

Much attention has focused on use of plasma from nontransfused male donors or female donors after fractionation.[7,11,12] Based on this data, the American Red Cross committed to implement this strategy of using male-predominant FP24 by late 2007. Availability issues, however, will likely limit use of only male-donated products.[13] Given the high volume of plasma required to adjust the INR and its documented unreliability in predicting bleeding diatheses in patients who have liver disease, prudent use of plasma, mainly in active hemorrhage when serum fibrinogen is low, is the best strategy to avoid sequelae such as TRALI.[3,14,15]

PLATELETS AND PACKED RED BLOOD CELLS

Based on work from Tripodi and colleagues[16] (see also the article by Tripodi elsewhere in this issue), increasing evidence provides guidance for using platelet transfusion in patients who have cirrhosis, although these important laboratory results require translation into the clinical setting. Based on work that focuses on endogenous thrombin production, adequate thrombin production seems to be present in cirrhosis when platelet counts are approximately 50,000 to 60,000/cc^3, whereas optimal levels are seen with levels of 100,000/cc^3 or more. Thus, based on current data, one could recommend platelet levels of at least 50,000/cc^3 for moderate-risk procedures (ie, liver biopsy) and closer to 100,000/cc^3 in very–high-risk procedures (ie, intracranial pressure monitor placement), although further investigation is needed to confirm these results in the clinical arena.

Red blood cell transfusion and its effects on pressures and intravascular volume are discussed further later. However, rheologic studies have indicated that normal platelet flow (at the periphery of the circulating blood stream where they are closer to potential binding sites in the event of vascular breach) is adversely affected with hematocrit levels less than 25%, supporting the recommendation to maintain this level in patients who have cirrhosis who are experiencing bleeding or about to undergo a high-risk procedure.[17–19]

Table 1	
Criteria for transfusion-related acute lung injury and transfusion-associated circulatory overload	
TRALI	**TACO**
Onset of symptoms within 6 h of transfusion	Onset of symptoms within 6 h of transfusion
Acute onset hypoxemia by conventional measures (A–a gradient >300 or room air SpO$_2$ <90%)	Acute onset hypoxemia by conventional measures (A–a gradient >300 or room air SpO$_2$ <90%)
Bilateral infiltrates	Bilateral infiltrates
Normal or low central venous pressure or pulmonary artery occlusion pressure	Presence of one of the following: pulmonary artery occlusion pressure ≥ 18 mm Hg; BNP >250 or pre-/posttransfusion BNP ratio ≥ 1.5; absence of rapid improvement with diuretic therapy
No underlying previous lung injury	Systolic EF <45% or systolic BP >160 mm Hg

Abbreviations: A–a gradient, alveolar–arterial gradient; BNP, serum brain natriuretic peptide; BP, blood pressure; EF, ejection fraction; SpO$_2$, oxygen saturation by pulse oximetry; TACO, transfusion-associated circulatory overload; TRALI, transfusion-related acute lung injury.

VOLUME EXPANSION, PORTAL HYPERTENSION, AND BLEEDING DIATHESIS IN CIRRHOSIS

The impact of volume expansion on renal function in patients who have chronic liver disease has been well-characterized in those who have undergone paracentesis and have hepatorenal syndrome.[20-23] However, the effects of volume expanders on systemic blood volume and portal circulation and subsequent risk for hemorrhage are more limited but suggest a role for a more conservative use of blood products. Prior studies have described a higher proportion of blood volume in the noncentral compartment, with portal circulatory pressures and renal arterial hemodynamic dysregulation increasing linearly with the severity of cirrhosis (**Fig. 2**).[24,25] Later analyses further focused these findings by showing increased filling of the splanchnic compartment related to portal hypertension in patients who had cirrhosis (**Fig. 3**).[26]

Effects on Portal Pressure

The relationship of variceal bleeding risk and portal hypertension is well documented.[27] A small number of studies address the portal effects of crystalloid infusion, plasma transfusion, or packed red cell transfusion in humans, but animal studies have explored portal circulatory changes after volume expansion, with interesting results favoring a more careful approach with volume expansion. The few existing human studies on the effect of crystalloid infusion on portal hemodynamics show that a mild transient increase in portal pressure ensues but that the final destination of these solutions is the interstitial space.[24]

In animal studies of blood transfusion, rats with more severe portal hypertension have more extreme increases in portal pressures with transfusion,[28] implying worsening vascular dysregulation as cirrhosis becomes more severe. Furthermore, rats with portal hypertension were subjected to controlled hemorrhage and then were transfused with 0%, 50%, or 100% of the volume of blood lost. The group that received 100% replacement had the lowest mean blood pressure, the highest rate of rebleeding, and the poorest overall survival.[29] Similarly, in humans who have cirrhosis, red cell transfusion leads to a linear increase in portal pressure,[30] which is blunted by administration of somatostatin.[31]

Concerning plasma transfusion, one early study showed that portal pressures in humans increased with plasma administration,[32] but no other human or animal study

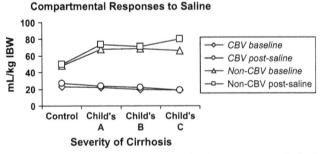

Fig. 2. Increasingly higher amounts of infused saline lead to proportionally higher expansion of the non–central blood volume as the severity of cirrhosis worsens. CBV, central blood volume; IBW, ideal body weight. (*Data from* Moller S, Bendtsen F, Henriksen JH. Effect of volume expansion on systemic hemodynamics and central and arterial blood volume in cirrhosis. Gastroenterology 1995;109:1917–25.)

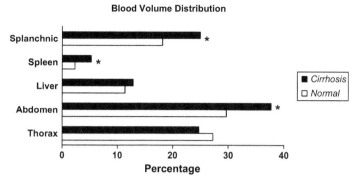

Fig. 3. The highest proportion of blood volume resides in the abdomen and specifically in the splanchnic circulation when compared with controls. Asterisk denotes a statistically significant difference in the distribution between groups. (*Data from* Kiszka-Kanowitz M, Henriksen JH, Moller S, et al. Blood volume distribution in patients with cirrhosis: aspects of the dual-head gamma-camera technique. J Hepatol 2001;35:605–12.)

seems to have specifically explored the effects of plasma on portal pressure in greater detail.

Use of plasma transfusion has led to higher red cell transfusion requirements in liver transplantation at a single European center,[33] but these results are hard to consider alone given that numerous factors affect transfusion needs in transplantation. Two additional human studies in patients who had cirrhosis showed that improved oxygen regulation after blood transfusion for anemia has beneficial homeostatic effects on portal vasomotor tone.[34,35] These findings support the hypotheses that plasma, in addition to its higher risk for TRALI, may provide fewer beneficial hemodynamic effects than blood transfusion and other volume expanders, with the caveat that overtransfusion after hemorrhage is likely harmful in patients who have cirrhosis.

Other Agents

Investigation of other volume expanders, including albumin, dextran, and hetastarch, has dramatically altered the standard of care for using these agents for specific indications in patients who have cirrhosis. Several studies successfully showed that administering albumin after large-volume paracentesis (LVP) decreased rates of renal failure by improving the effective arterial volume through modulation of the renin-angiotensin-aldosterone system (RAAS) and not through changes in portal pressures.[21,36,37] These trials confirmed earlier work showing no differences in the changes in portal pressure parameters after LVP between patients receiving albumin and those who did not, with both experiencing slight increases in portal pressure.[38] Patients receiving albumin after LVP had far less change in renal artery pressures, whereas those not receiving albumin had substantial renal arterial vasoconstriction and activation of renin and aldosterone production (**Fig. 4**). Albumin probably benefits patients who have cirrhosis by positively impacting vasomotor tone through additional pleiotropic effects, many of which likely involve its function as an intravascular transporter or scavenger of toxic molecules and intermediates (**Box 1**).[39]

Investigation of the effects of dextran, hetastarch, and hemaccel in patients who have cirrhosis has focused mainly on arterial effects; their portal effects are unclear. None of the agents is as consistently effective as albumin in preventing renal failure after large volume paracentesis.[40–43] The effects of colloid agents on hemostasis

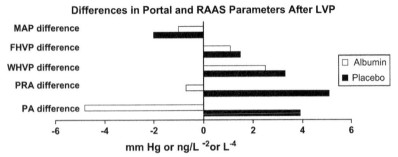

Fig. 4. Systemic and portal circulatory parameters change similarly in patients who have cirrhosis after large-volume paracentesis regardless of albumin infusion. The renin-angiotensin-aldosterone system, however, is activated in patients who have cirrhosis who did not receive albumin, but seems to be suppressed by albumin administration. (*Data from* Luca A, Garcia-Pagan JC, Bosch J, et al. Beneficial effects of intravenous albumin infusion on the hemodynamic and humoral changes after total paracentesis. Hepatology 1995;22:753–8; with permission.)

are relatively small, except with extreme hemodilution (loss of approximately 30%–40% of total blood volume). In vitro and in vivo studies using automated whole-blood clotting assays and thromboelastography show that dextran and hetastarch clearly have net anticoagulant effects, probably mediated by mild to moderate inhibition of platelet aggregation and adhesion, although the clinical significance of these effects is likely minor.[44–48]

COAGULOPATHY AND RENAL FAILURE IN PATIENTS WHO HAVE CIRRHOSIS

Acute kidney injury (AKI) frequently occurs in patients who have cirrhosis experiencing an acute decompensation in liver function. Hepatorenal syndrome (HRS) is a leading

---

Box 1
Potential nononcotic effects of albumin

Intravascular transport

Depot function and transporter of numerous metabolites

Binds and interacts with numerous drugs

Scavenging

Thiols scavenge reactive oxygen and nitrogen species

Binds copper, which is a known accelerant of reactive oxygen species generation

Anti-inflammatory effects

Binds arachidonic acid, which increases capillary permeability

Interferes with xanthine oxidase-mediated neutrophil adhesion

Reduces inflammation resulting from endotoxemia

Stems neutrophil oxidative burst in response to inflammatory cytokines

Redox regulation may influence transcription factor activity in systemic inflammatory states

Anticoagulant effects

Thiols bind nitric oxide, thus prolonging nitric oxide's inhibitory effects on platelet aggregation

cause of AKI in these patients, but other causes may coexist, some of which may be reversible without liver transplantation.[21,49] The associated morbidity and mortality rates are very high in these situations, and various forms of extracorporeal or renal replacement therapies (RRT) are used either as a bridge therapy while awaiting liver transplantation or as a temporizing measure if the cause of AKI is potentially reversible. Currently no definitive evidence exists of improved long-term outcomes with institution of hemodialysis or extracorporeal liver-assist devices in patients who have cirrhosis and AKI.[49] When needed, conventional hemodialysis is the most frequently used RRT in patients who have cirrhosis. Critically ill patients frequently have associated hemodynamic instability that requires use of a continuous hemodialysis modality. Selected renal replacement therapies include conventional hemodialysis continuous renal replacement therapies, including continuous venovenous hemofiltration, continuous venovenous hemodialysis, and continuous venovenous hemodiafiltration; extracorporeal albumin dialysis (molecular adsorbent recirculation system [MARS]); and Prometheus.

Conventional Hemodialysis
Continuous Renal Replacement Therapies
    Continuous venovenous hemofiltration (CVVH)
    Continuous venovenous hemodialysis (CVVHD)
    Continuous venovenous hemodiafiltration (CVVHDF)
Extracorporeal Albumin Dialysis (Molecular Adsorbent Recirculating System (MARS))
Prometheus

Hemodialysis is helpful in many indications in patients who have cirrhosis, especially in providing net ultrafiltration to prevent development of pulmonary edema and need for intensive care while the liver transplantation evaluation process is ongoing. Common indications for renal replacement therapies in patients who have cirrhosis include:

Severe fluid overload
Severe hyperkalemia
Severe metabolic acidosis
Severe azotemia (usually with suspicion of uremia)
Acute intoxications (drugs)
Failure of other pharmacologic/nonpharmacologic interventions
Type II hepatorenal syndrome
Novel extracorporeal/renal replacement therapies (eg, MARS, Prometheus)

Coagulation abnormalities are common in patients who have AKI, but few studies have specifically examined coagulopathy and platelet function in those who have cirrhosis with AKI. The characteristic defects seen in patients who have renal failure are likely amplified in those who have cirrhosis because of underlying thrombocytopenia and variable coagulation factor levels and effectiveness.

Uremic Platelet Dysfunction

Platelet dysfunction in uremia is a well-established, multifactorial phenomenon that chiefly involves abnormalities in platelet adhesion and the interaction between platelets and endothelium.[50] Granules in platelets from patients who have uremia function poorly, and toxins such as urea, creatinine, and phenols also negatively affect platelet aggregation by decreasing von Willebrand's factor and fibrinogen binding to glycoprotein IIb/IIIa.[51] Functional platelets become dysfunctional in uremic plasma, and the function of uremic platelets is partially corrected when placed in nonuremic plasma. Activation of coagulation and fibrinolysis after platelet degranulation also possibly plays a role.[52] Several cytoskeletal deficiencies in patients who have uremia impair platelet contraction and thus lead to decreased platelet mobility and secretory function.[53] Nitric oxide and its associated mediators are increased in patients who have renal failure, which weaken platelet–platelet and platelet–endothelium interactions.[51]

Dialysis Catheter Placement

Central catheter placement for RRT in patients who have cirrhosis is a common procedure, yet few data are available to provide guidance for appropriate use of prophylactic blood products to prevent bleeding complications.[54] Studies of bleeding complications of central vein catheterization in patients who have abnormal prothrombin time PT/INR who did not receive preprocedure blood products describe very low complication rates, ranging from 0% to 0.2%, with most patients also having abnormal platelet counts.[55–57]

Prospective studies of complications of femoral-based arteriography in patients who had similar abnormalities in their PT and platelet counts showed complication rates ranging from 0% to 1.2% without pretreatment, which were comparable to rates in patients who underwent normal laboratory evaluation.[58–60] These data suggest that venous and arterial catheterization is safe in patients who have abnormal coagulation parameters and that preprocedure blood products are rarely needed. Among the most severely ill patients who had cirrhosis in a study of the MARS extracorporeal liver-assist device, 21% experienced central venous catheter site bleeding before use of MARS, and an additional 6% had further catheter site bleeding.[61]

Renal Replacement Therapy

Use of conventional or continuous RRT in AKI has specific effects on coagulation, mostly tending toward hypercoagulability, although it is largely subclinical in nature. Turbulence and shear occurring during RRT lead to platelet activation. Platelets can bind fibrinogen adherent to the artificial surface during low flow periods by way of the GPIIb/IIIa receptor. Thrombin formation and GPIIb/IIIa receptor activation lead to platelet degranulation, platelet aggregation, and activation of the coagulation mechanism. Contact activation also occurs with leukocytes, including degranulation causing coaggregation of platelets and white cells, which express tissue factor, and resultant coagulation activation.[62]

In addition to cellular and platelet activation, contact of blood on artificial surfaces of the circuit can occur through intrinsic pathway mechanisms, which mainly rely on factor XIIa concentrations and blood flow. Air traps also operate under low flow, leading to air–blood interfaces and turbulence, with ensuing induction of coagulation.[63] These procoagulant changes may be somewhat offset by worsening of thrombocytopenia during hemodialysis secondary to complement activation induced by contact of blood components with the dialyzer's bioartificial membrane.[51]

Despite the perceived elevated risk for bleeding, anticoagulation techniques are often needed to prevent the thrombotic dysfunction of the extracorporeal circuit.[62] Using regional anticoagulation techniques using citrate minimizes additional risk to patients who have cirrhosis.[64] Citrate inhibits coagulation in the circuit by chelating magnesium and calcium. Because citrate is metabolized by the liver and has a high sodium content, acid–base abnormalities or inefficient ultrafiltration may occur in patients who have cirrhosis, which may require customization of the dialysate makeup. Citrate anticoagulation in hemodialysis has unique advantages over traditional anticoagulants in reducing the risk for induced bleeding diatheses through limiting blood deposits on the biomembrane and improving biocompatibility.[65] These improvements with citrate anticoagulation may be significant in patients who have liver disease, in whom bleeding tendencies may be hard to assess.[63]

Other novel alternatives include extracorporeal therapies with specialized focus on patients who have liver disease (eg, ELAD, MARS, Prometheus).[66–68] Many of the extracorporeal therapies used in combined liver and kidney failure have been tested in small clinical trials with promising results. Platelet and coagulation effects of these intensive assist devices present similar thrombotic issues because of the use of an extracorporeal circuit.[69]

VOLUME CONTRACTION THERAPY

Despite increased experience and improvements in surgical technique, packed red cell transfusion still occurs frequently with liver transplantation and negatively impacts outcomes of liver transplantation.[70] Active reduction in blood volume using phlebotomy and other volume control measures is a new strategy in preliminary stages of investigation to minimize bleeding risk in critically ill patients who have cirrhosis. The highest quality data supporting this practice are from a study in which plasma avoidance and maintenance of a low central venous pressure with phlebotomy minimized red cell transfusion requirements and improved survival in 100 consecutive liver transplantations compared with standard management.[71] This technique is developing an enthusiastic following among transplant surgeons (see article by Porte and colleagues elsewhere in this volume) and may carry implications for managing patients who have decompensated cirrhosis and warrants further research.

SUMMARY

Plasma-based products are commonly used in patients who have chronic liver disease despite sparse clinical evidence of its efficacy in meaningfully altering coagulation. This maneuver is fraught with potentially devastating risks, including TRALI. Steps are being taken to reduce its incidence, but selective use of plasma in patients who have chronic liver disease is likely the best course of action. However, volume expansion is often required in the care of patients who have cirrhosis related to hemorrhage or systemic infection. Crystalloid infusion only temporarily provides blood volume expansion in patients who have cirrhosis, and red cell transfusions may have several detrimental effects if overused.

Plasma-based therapy has undergone only cursory controlled investigation, and several theoretic and proven situational disadvantages should limit its use in patients who have cirrhosis for correcting the INR. Albumin is probably the most effective of these, because it has shown benefit in maintaining renovascular homeostasis while having minimal effects on portal hemodynamics and hemostasis. Alternative volume expanders have not been as effective as albumin and confer slightly higher risks for bleeding complications but cost significantly less.

Renal replacement therapies are frequent adjuncts in the care of patients who have cirrhosis with acute decompensation or who require bridge therapy to liver transplantation. Novel extracorporeal therapies show much promise but have not yet been shown to consistently alter survival in acute-on-chronic liver failure. Numerous pro- and anticoagulant effects occur with use of RRT and extracorporeal liver-assist therapy, and the net effect on coagulopathy in patients who have cirrhosis with AKI is unclear.

Volume contraction is a new area of investigation of coagulopathy-related therapies. This practice involves active maintenance of a low central venous pressure using phlebotomy and judicious volume management. It has shown promising initial results and merits further evaluation as a feasible strategy in managing patients who have cirrhosis.

REFERENCES

1. Stanworth SJ, Brunskill SJ, Hyde CJ, et al. Is fresh frozen plasma clinically effective? Br J Haematol 2004;126:139–52.
2. Holland L, Sarode R. Should plasma be transfused prophylactically before invasive procedures? Curr Opin Hematol 2006;13:447–51.
3. Holland LL, Brooks JP. Toward rational fresh frozen plasma transfusion: the effect of plasma transfusion on coagulation test results. Am J Clin Pathol 2006;126:1–7.
4. Bux J, Sachs UJ. The pathogenesis of transfusion-related acute lung injury (TRALI). Br J Haematol 2007;136:788–99.
5. Kleinman S, Caulfield T, Chan P, et al. Toward an understanding of transfusion-related acute lung injury: statement of a consensus panel. Transfusion 2004;44: 1774–89.
6. Khan H, Belsher J, Yilmaz M, et al. Fresh-frozen plasma and platelet transfusions are associated with development of acute lung injury in critically ill medical patients. Chest 2007;131:1308–14.
7. Eder AF, Herron R, Strupp A, et al. Transfusion-related acute lung injury surveillance (2003–2005) and the potential impact of the selective use of plasma from male donors in the American Red Cross. Transfusion 2007;47:599–607.
8. Gajic O, Rana R, Winters JL, et al. Transfusion-related acute lung injury in the critically ill: prospective nested case-control study. Am J Respir Crit Care Med 2007;176:886–91.
9. Rana R, Fernández-Pérez ER, Khan SA, et al. Transfusion-related acute lung injury and pulmonary edema in critically ill patients: a retrospective study. Transfusion 2006;46:1478–83.
10. Skeate RC, Eastlund T. Distinguishing between transfusion related acute lung injury and transfusion associated circulatory overload. Curr Opin Hematol 2007;14: 682–7.
11. Gajic O, Yilmaz M, Iscimen R, et al. Transfusion from male-only versus female donors in critically ill recipients of high plasma volume components. Crit Care Med 2007;35:1645–8.
12. Silliman CC. High-volume transfusion from male-only versus female donor plasma and hypoxemia in the critically ill. Crit Care Med 2007;35:1775.
13. Benjamin R. Transfusion-related acute lung injury (TRALI): immunologic issues regarding donors and patients. In: American Society for Apheresis Annual Meeting. 2006;Las Vegas (NV). Available at: http://www.apheresis.org/%7EDOCUMENTS/Wed_0815.5_Benjamin_Venetian_BC.pdf. Accessed December 12, 2007.
14. MacLennan S, Barbara JA. Risks and side effects of therapy with plasma and plasma fractions. Baillieres Best Pract Res Clin Haematol 2006;19:169–89.
15. Tripodi A, Caldwell SH, Hoffman M, et al. Review article: the prothrombin time test as a measure of bleeding risk and prognosis in liver disease. Aliment Pharmacol Ther 2007;26:141–8.
16. Tripodi A, Primignani M, Chantarangkul V, et al. Thrombin generation in patients with cirrhosis: the role of platelets. Hepatology 2006;44:440–5.
17. Bergqvist D, Arfors KE. The effect of normovolemic hemodilution on microvascular hemostasis in the rabbit. Res Exp Med 1979;175:61–6.

18. Turitto VT, Weiss HJ. Red blood cells: their dual role in thrombus formation. Science 1980;207:541–3.
19. Hathcock JJ. Flow effects on coagulation and thrombosis. Arterioscler Thromb Vasc Biol 2006;26:1729–37.
20. Gines P, Tito L, Arroyo V, et al. Randomized comparative study of therapeutic paracentesis with and without intravenous albumin in cirrhosis. Gastroenterology 1988;94:1493–502.
21. Gines A, Escorsell A, Gines P, et al. Incidence, predictive factors, and prognosis of the hepatorenal syndrome in cirrhosis with ascites. Gastroenterology 1993; 105:229–36.
22. Sort P, Navasa M, Arroyo V, et al. Effect of intravenous albumin on renal impairment and mortality in patients with cirrhosis and spontaneous bacterial peritonitis. N Engl J Med 1999;341:403–9.
23. Ortega R, Gines P, Uriz J, et al. Terlipressin therapy with and without albumin for patients with hepatorenal syndrome: results of a prospective, nonrandomized study. Hepatology 2002;36(4 Pt 1):941–8.
24. Hadengue A, Moreau R, Gaudin C, et al. Total effective vascular compliance in patients with cirrhosis: a study of the response to acute blood volume expansion. Hepatology 1992;15:809–15.
25. Moller S, Bendtsen F, Henriksen JH. Effect of volume expansion on systemic hemodynamics and central and arterial blood volume in cirrhosis. Gastroenterology 1995;109:1917–25.
26. Kiszka-Kanowitz M, Henriksen JH, Moller S, et al. Blood volume distribution in patients with cirrhosis: aspects of the dual-head gamma-camera technique. J Hepatol 2001;35:605–12.
27. D'Amico G, Garcia-Pagan JC, Luca A, et al. Hepatic vein pressure gradient reduction and prevention of variceal bleeding in cirrhosis: a systematic review. Gastroenterology 2006;131:1611–24.
28. Kravetz D, Bosch J, Arderiu M, et al. Hemodynamic effects of blood volume restitution following a hemorrhage in rats with portal hypertension due to cirrhosis of the liver: influence of the extent of portal-systemic shunting. Hepatology 1989;9:808–14.
29. Castaneda B, Morales J, Lionetti R, et al. Effects of blood volume restitution following a portal hypertensive-related bleeding in anesthetized cirrhotic rats. Hepatology 2001;33:821–5.
30. Zimmon DS, Kessler RE. The portal pressure-blood volume relationship in cirrhosis. Gut 1974;15:99–101.
31. Villanueva C, Ortiz J, Minana J, et al. Somatostatin treatment and risk stratification by continuous portal pressure monitoring during acute variceal bleeding. Gastroenterology 2001;121:110–7.
32. Boyer JL, Chatterjee C, Iber FL, et al. Effect of plasma-volume expansion on portal hypertension. N Engl J Med 1966;275:750–5.
33. Massicotte L, Sassine M-P, Lenis S, et al. Transfusion predictors in liver transplant. Anesth Analg 2004;98:1245–51.
34. Cirera I, Elizalde JI, Pique JM, et al. Anemia worsens hyperdynamic circulation of patients with cirrhosis and portal hypertension. Dig Dis Sci 1997;42:1697–702.
35. Elizalde JI, Moitinho E, Garcia-Pagan JC, et al. Effects of increasing blood hemoglobin levels on systemic hemodynamics of acutely anemic cirrhotic patients. J Hepatol 1998;29:789–95.
36. Tito L, Gines P, Arroyo V, et al. Total paracentesis associated with intravenous albumin management of patients with cirrhosis and ascites. Gastroenterology 1990;98:146–51.

37. Garcia-Compean D, Zacarias Villarreal J, Bahena Cuevas H, et al. Total therapeutic paracentesis (TTP) with and without intravenous albumin in the treatment of cirrhotic tense ascites: a randomized controlled trial. Liver 1993;13: 233–8.
38. Luca A, Garcia-Pagan JC, Bosch J, et al. Beneficial effects of intravenous albumin infusion on the hemodynamic and humoral changes after total paracentesis. Hepatology 1995;22:753–8.
39. Evans TW. Albumin as a drug—biological effects of albumin unrelated to oncotic pressure. Aliment Pharmacol Ther 2002;16(Suppl 5):6–11.
40. Planas R, Gines P, Arroyo V, et al. Dextran-70 versus albumin as plasma expanders in cirrhotic patients with tense ascites treated with total paracentesis. Results of a randomized study. Gastroenterology 1990;99:1736–44.
41. Fassio E, Terg R, Landeira G, et al. Paracentesis with Dextran 70 vs. paracentesis with albumin in cirrhosis with tense ascites. J Hepatol 1992;14(2–3):310–6.
42. Sola R, Vila MC, Andreu M, et al. Total paracentesis with dextran 40 vs diuretics in the treatment of ascites in cirrhosis: a randomized controlled study. J Hepatol 1994;20:282–8.
43. Gines A, Fernandez-Esparrach G, Monescillo A, et al. Randomized trial comparing albumin, dextran 70, and polygeline in cirrhotic patients with ascites treated by paracentesis. Gastroenterology 1996;111:1002–10.
44. Van der Linden P, Ickx BE. The effects of colloid solutions on hemostasis. Can J Anaesth 2006;53(Suppl 6):S30–9.
45. Jones SB, Whitten CW, Despotis GJ, et al. The influence of crystalloid and colloid replacement solutions in acute normovolemic hemodilution: a preliminary survey of hemostatic markers. Anesth Analg 2003;96:363–8.
46. Ekseth K, Abildgaard L, Vegfors M, et al. The in vitro effects of crystalloids and colloids on coagulation. Anaesthesia 2002;57:1102–8.
47. de Jonge E, Levi M. Effects of different plasma substitutes on blood coagulation: a comparative review. Crit Care Med 2001;29:1261–7.
48. Mortier E, Ongenae M, De Baerdemaeker L, et al. In vitro evaluation of the effect of profound haemodilution with hydroxyethyl starch 6%, modified fluid gelatin 4% and dextran 40 10% on coagulation profile measured by thromboelastography. Anaesthesia 1997;52:1061–4.
49. Wadei HM, Mai ML, Ahsan N, et al. Hepatorenal syndrome: pathophysiology and management. Clin J Am Soc Nephrol 2006;1:1066–79.
50. Kaw D, Malhotra D. Platelet dysfunction and end-stage renal disease. Semin Dial 2006;19:317–22.
51. Boccardo P, Remuzzi G, Galbusera M. Platelet dysfunction in renal failure. Semin Thromb Hemost 2004;30:579–89.
52. Mezzano D, Tagle R, Panes O. Hemostatic disorder of uremia: the platelet defect, the main determinant of prolonged bleeding time, is correlated with indices of activation of coagulation and fibrinolysis. Thromb Haemost 1996;76:312–21.
53. Escolar G, Diaz-Ricart M, Cases A. Abnormal cytoskeletal assembly in platelets from uremic patients. Am J Pathol 1991;143:823–31.
54. Segal JH, Dzik WH. Paucity of studies to support that abnormal coagulation test results predict bleeding in the setting of invasive procedures. Transfusion 2005; 45:1413–25.
55. Fisher NC, Mutimer DJ. Central venous cannulation in patients with liver disease and coagulopathy—a prospective audit. Intensive Care Med 1999;25:481–5.
56. Foster PF, Moore LR, Sankary HN, et al. Central venous catheterization in patients with coagulopathy. Arch Surg 1992;127:273–5.

57. Doerfler ME, Kaufman B, Goldenberg AS. Central venous catheter placement in patients with disorders of hemostasis. Chest 1996;110:185–8.

58. Wilson NV, Corne JM, Given-Wilson RM. A critical appraisal of coagulation studies prior to transfemoral angiography. Br J Radiol 1990;63:147–8.

59. Darcy MD, Kanterman RY, Kleinhoffer MA, et al. Evaluation of coagulation tests as predictors of angiographic bleeding. Radiology 1996;198:741–4.

60. MacDonald LA, Beohar N, Wang NC, et al. A comparison of arterial closure devices to manual compression in liver transplantation candidates undergoing coronary angiography. J Invasive Cardiol 2003;15:1568–70.

61. Faybik P, Bacher A, Kozek-Langenecker SA, et al. Molecular adsorbent recirculating system and hemostasis in patients at high risk of bleeding: an observational study. Crit Care 2006;10(1):R24.

62. Northup PG, Sundaram V, Fallon MB, et al. Hypercoagulation and thrombophilia in liver disease. J Thromb Haemost 2008;6(1):2–9.

63. Fischer KG. Essentials of anticoagulation in hemodialysis. Hemodial Int 2007;11: 178–89.

64. Vargas Hein O, Kox WJ, Spies C. Anticoagulation in continuous renal replacement therapy. Contrib Nephrol 2004;144:308–16.

65. Hofbauer R, Moser D, Frass M, et al. Effect of anticoagulation on blood membrane interactions during hemodialysis. Kidney Int 1999;56:1578–83.

66. Mitzner SR, Stange J, Klammt S, et al. Extracorporeal detoxification using the molecular adsorbent recirculating system for critically ill patients with liver failure. J Am Soc Nephrol 2001;12(Suppl 17):S75–82.

67. Rifai K, Ernst T, Kretschmer U, et al. Prometheus—a new extracorporeal system for the treatment of liver failure. J Hepatol 2003;39:984–90.

68. Rifai K, Tetta C, Ronco C. Prometheus: from legend to the real liver support therapy. Int J Artif Organs 2007;30:858–63.

69. Pryor HI II, Vacanti JP. The promise of artificial liver replacement. Front Biosci 2008;13:2140–59.

70. Ramos E, Dalmau A, Sabate A, et al. Intraoperative red blood cell transfusion in liver transplantation: influence on patient outcome, prediction of requirements, and measures to reduce them. Liver Transpl 2003;9:1320–7.

71. Massicotte L, Lenis S, Thibeault L, et al. Effect of low central venous pressure and phlebotomy on blood product transfusion requirements during liver transplantations. Liver Transpl 2006;12:117–23.

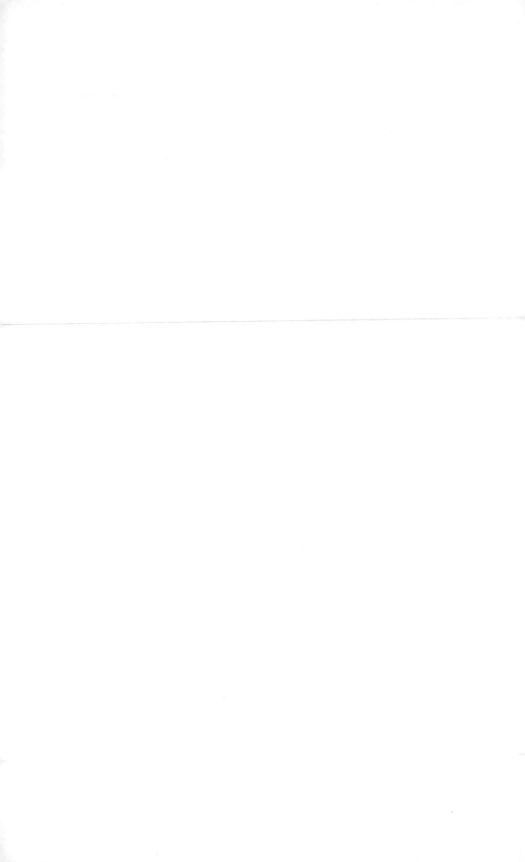

The Role of Anti-Fibrinolytics, rFVIIa and Other Pro-Coagulants: Prophylactic Versus Rescue?

Neeral L. Shah, MD*, Stephen H. Caldwell, MD, Carl L. Berg, MD

KEYWORDS

- Recombinant factor VIIa • Anti-fibrinolytics • Bleeding risk
- Prophylactic therapy • Rescue therapy

Patients who have end-stage liver disease often undergo procedures that have a risk for significant bleeding and complications. Therefore, therapies to prevent and treat bleeding in the setting of liver disease should be an important aspect of clinical management. This article discusses two products that are currently used to treat active bleeding or decrease the bleeding risk in patients who have severe liver disease. First, recombinant factor VIIa (rFVIIa), which is the activated form of factor VII (FVII), can facilitate clot formation through amplifying the thrombin burst and accentuation of platelet function. Second, although the exact prevalence of hyperfibrinolysis in liver disease remains uncertain, antifibrinolytic therapy can be used to decrease the rate of clot lysis. However, the controversy regarding interpretation of conventional tests of coagulation in cirrhosis (see article by Tripodi elsewhere in this issue) extends into the field of therapeutics. For example, is it sufficient to correct the international normalized ratio (INR) before an invasive procedure in a patient who has liver disease or do the inherent limitations of this test likewise render the test an invalid end point? Many of these questions have not been resolved. This article reviews the current literature regarding rFVIIa and anti-fibrinolytic therapy in liver disease.

RECOMBINANT ACTIVATED FACTOR VIIA

rFVIIa was developed in the late 1990s to treat hemophiliacs.[1] The first reported use of activated factor VII (FVIIa) was during an open knee joint operation on a hemophiliac.[2]

Division of Gastroenterology and Hepatology, West Complex Box 800708, Department of Gastroenterology and Hepatology, University of Virginia, Charlottesville, VA 22908, USA
* Corresponding author.
E-mail address: neeral.shah@virginia.edu (N.L. Shah).

Clin Liver Dis 13 (2009) 87–93
doi:10.1016/j.cld.2008.09.005
1089-3261/08/$ – see front matter © 2009 Elsevier Inc. All rights reserved.
liver.theclinics.com

This drastically changed management because it reduced bleeding in procedures that were previously contraindicated in these patients. It has been used recently in various disease processes, including cirrhosis, as a treatment and prophylaxis of bleeding. Clearly, FVIIa plays an important role in normal coagulation, because it regulates the initial set of reactions toward clot formation that occurs at a site of vascular breach (for additional details, see the article by Monroe and Hoffman elsewhere in this issue).[3] However, its use in liver disease has been more difficult to establish and remains controversial, largely because of its high cost and some risk for thrombotic complications, although most studies (reviewed later) have been encouraging.

Bernstein and colleagues[4] reported one of the first investigations of patients who had cirrhosis in 1997. In this study, the group aimed to prove that prothrombin times could be reduced in nonbleeding patients who had cirrhosis. The sample population consisted of 10 patients who had prothrombin times greater than 2 seconds above the upper limit of normal. The study lasted 10 days, and subjects received three injections of rFVIIa. The patients received a graduated dose of rFVIIa, starting with 5 μg/kg, then 20 μg/kg, and finally 80 μg/kg. This study showed a statistically significant dose-dependent effect with normalization of the prothrombin time after the injections for 2, 6, and 12 hours, respectively.

In 2002, Jeffers and colleagues[5] reported on the use of four different doses of rFVIIa; 5, 20, 80, and 120 μg/kg in a randomized, double-blind, controlled trial of 66 patients undergoing laparoscopic liver biopsies. The results showed that 74% of patients experienced hemostasis (measured as the laparoscopically observed liver bleeding time) within the first 10 minutes of the injection. None required transfusions or additional intervention for bleeding. However, consistent with limitations of conventional assays, the observed liver bleeding time showed no correlation to correction of the measured prothrombin time. One patient was noted to have portal vein thrombosis attributed to underlying liver disease, and one subsequent episode of disseminated intravascular coagulation was noted but also attributed to advanced liver failure and multiorgan failure.

Bosch and colleagues[6] studied the use of rFVIIa in 242 patients who had cirrhosis and active upper gastrointestinal bleeding. These patients were randomized to two arms; placebo and eight doses of 100 μg/kg of rFVIIa. The intervention was given as an adjunct to standard care to help achieve hemostasis. The study found a significant difference using a composite end point but benefit was seen only in those patients who had advanced (Child-Pugh class C) liver disease. Their experience was also supported by an uncontrolled series reported by Romero-Castro and colleagues[7] in 2004 on the use of FVIIa in eight patients who had severe variceal hemorrhage. The patients were eligible for the study if they were nonresponsive to endoscopic or pharmacologic therapy or to balloon tamponade. Each of these patients was given a single dose of 4.8 mg of rFVIIa, and all experienced hemostasis.

A second study by Bosch and colleagues[8] currently in press, compares the use of low- and high-dose rFVIIa to control bleeding in patients who had advanced cirrhosis with active variceal bleeding. The results showed no difference in controlling bleeding within the first 24 hours and no difference in rebleeding or mortality rates at day 5. The only statistically significant secondary end point was a lower mortality rate at 42 days for the group who received high-dose rFVIIa. However, the very high doses (and associated costs) noted in the Bosch studies coupled with the limited, albeit positive results in subset analysis, reduce the likelihood that rFVIIa will find a role in the routine management of variceal bleeding, although it may have a significant role as a rescue agent (discussed later).

Further studies investigated the use of rFVIIa in patients who had fulminant liver failure and those needing liver transplantation.[9,10] In a retrospective cohort study at the University of Virginia, eight patients who experienced fulminant hepatic failure who received fresh frozen plasma (FFP) alone as prophylaxis for intracranial pressure monitor placement were compared with seven patients who received less FFP and rFVIIa (40 μg/kg) with an aim to correcting the prolonged INR. Those who received FFP alone had no correction of the INR; however, all patients receiving rFVIIa achieved normal INR. Overall, the patients receiving rFVIIa had more expedited completion of high-risk procedures and significantly less anasarca; however, no difference was seen in bleeding complications, survival, or rates of transplantation.

Two studies in 2005 reported on the effect of preoperative or perioperative administration of rFVIIa with liver transplantation. The first study involved a single infusion of rFVIIa before proceeding to transplantation at three different doses; 20, 40, and 80 μg/kg.[11] This technique provided transient correction of the prolonged prothrombin time, but the effect was short-lived and again the significance of correcting this test result remains questionable. The half-life of a single dose of rFVIIa in this setting was estimated to be approximately 2.89 hours in stable patients and 2.3 hours in bleeding patients.[12] The other study repeated infusions every 2 hours until 30 minutes before graft reperfusion.[13] This approach maintained conventional coagulation indices closer to normal, but, consistent with the limitations of conventional tests in predicting bleeding, did not reduce the patient's transfusion need.

Although rFVIIa has clearly shown efficacy in correcting the prothrombin time and INR, it has been more difficult to show a clear reduction in bleeding risk. This situation probably more reflects deficiencies of the target tests, such as INR in liver disease (see article by Tripodi elsewhere in this issue), rather than lack of efficacy of the agent, given its in vitro effects and even augmentation of platelet function.[14] Clearly, further studies are warranted to investigate the agent in patients stratified by more accurate measures of bleeding risk, such as may be offered by the endogenous thrombin production (ETP) test or thromboelastography. Complications of rFVIIa are infrequent but not surprisingly include the risk for thrombotic events. Cost also remains a significant concern; a typical adult dose at 40 μg/kg costs $4000 to $6000.[15]

ANTIFIBRINOLYTIC DRUGS

Inhibition of clot lysis is another approach to promoting hemostasis. Derivatives of the amino acid lysine, 6-amnohexanoic acid (aminocaproic acid) and 4-(aminomethyl) cyclohexanecarboyxylic acid (tranexamic acid), are grouped in the class of medications named *antifibrinolytics*. Another variant of these medications is aprotinin, a serine protease inhibitor. Plasmin, a protein responsible for fibrinolysis and fibrin degradation, is the active form of its precursor, plasminogen. Direct inhibition of plasmin is one mechanism of the serine protease inhibitor aprotinin. Furthermore, the conversion to plasmin only occurs if plasminogen is bound to fibrin at a lysine receptor site. Through competitive inhibition, the lysine-derivative antifibrinolytics—aminocaproic and tranexamic acids—prevent plasmin formation. Thus, by differing mechanisms, aminocaproic acid, tranexamic acid, and aprotinin reduce fibrinolysis and prevent clot destruction.

These agents may be especially appropriate when hyperfibrinolysis (see article by Ferro and colleagues elsewhere in this issue) or dysfibrinogenemia is known or suspected. The presence of hyperfibrinolysis, although evident on tests such as thromboelastography, is much more difficult to diagnose by conventional assays like prothrombin time or INR, which can be near normal. Hyperfibrinolysis or dysfibrinogenemia should be suspected in the presence of mucosal (gum) bleeding or late bleeding (such as hours postbiopsy or line placement), suggesting that clot has formed and prematurely dissolved. Most body cavity fluids, such as saliva, ascites, and urine, possess fibrinolytic capacity, and thus bleeding in these areas may be especially amenable to this approach.

Antifibrinolytics have been used in the clinical setting of primary menorrhagia, upper gastrointestinal bleeding, dental extractions in patients who have coagulopathies, and bleeding associated with thrombocytopenia.[16] Patients who have liver disease possess their own unique factors that lead to an increased rate of fibrinolysis and clot breakdown. First, these patients have an increased concentration of tissue plasminogen activator because of decreased hepatic clearance. Second, hepatic production of a fibrinolysis inhibitor, thrombin activatable fibrinolysis inhibitor, is decreased from liver cirrhosis. Finally, a decreased concentration of α-2 antiplasmin, an inhibitor to plasmin activity, is also noted in patients who have cirrhosis.[17]

Numerous studies have examined the use of aprotinin to diminish hemorrhage in the setting of major surgery.[18,19] As shown by these studies, most of which have involved cardiac surgery, aprotinin has proven success in the perioperative setting to reduce bleeding and transfusion requirements. Much fewer data are established in patients who have liver disease. During liver transplantation, an increased fibrinolysis state occurs, especially at hepatic revascularization. Theoretically, the use of antifibrinolytics should attenuate the level of this fibrinolysis state and decrease bleeding risk.[16] The first study involving orthotopic liver transplantation in 2000 showed reduced blood transfusion requirements in patients receiving perioperative aprotinin.[20] Aprotinin was given 20 minutes before the surgery and was continued intraoperatively as an infusion until 2 hours after graft reperfusion. The aprotinin dosage was split between high- and regular-dose groups. These groups showed a significant reduction in blood transfusions by 37% and 20%, respectively.

However, other studies show no statistical difference in bleeding risk with the administration of aprotinin or placebo.[21] For this reason, some controversy still exists regarding its use. This conundrum may again result from inadequate risk stratification of patients who have liver disease who may have various bleeding diatheses, some appropriately managed by a particular treatment, but none adequately defined by conventional coagulation indices such as the INR.

The lysine derivatives, aminocaproic acid and tranexamic acid, are even less well studied in patients who have liver disease. However, aminocaproic acid has been shown to reduce fibrinolysis and possibly decrease active bleeding. One study examining 37 patients who had cirrhosis with soft tissue and subcutaneous bleeding showed more than 90% resolution of bleeding after the use of aminocaproic acid in the setting of hyperfibrinolysis.[17] However, when compared directly to tranexamic acid, aminocaproic acid did not have as significant an effect on blood transfusion requirements during orthotopic liver transplantation.[22] Aside from limited studies and uncertain therapeutic targets, several problems exist in interpreting the existing literature on these agents. Most problematic is that the doses of the antifibrinolytics vary significantly from among studies. Thus, reported doses in noncirrhosis studies include tranexamic acid given anywhere from 3 to 10 g, with a loading dose ranging from 2 to 7 g. Similarly, aminocaproic acid has been used over a wide range of dosing with an average total dose of 10 to 30 g, and a loading dose ranging from 1 to 15 g.[23] These wide ranges further indicate the need for clinical research to define the most appropriate doses and targets of therapy in patients who have liver disease.

All antifibrinolytics are associated with increased risk for thrombosis. Case reports describe thrombotic complications involving pulmonary, hepatic, and graft vasculature during transplantation. Aprotinin is also noted to have an increased risk for renal failure and hypersensitivity. This protein, derived from porcine lung tissue, can cause an allergic reaction consisting of a rash, urticaria, itching, and a histamine release leading to hypotension.[19] Tranexamic acid is well tolerated, but has reportedly caused episodes of nausea and gastrointestinal symptoms. Finally, aminocaproic acid has been described to cause renal dysfunction and skeletal muscle weakness. Nonetheless, their judicious use in patients who have liver disease may be especially beneficial with bleeding into body cavities where fibrinolytic activity may be especially high, such as postdental extraction bleeding,[24] hemothorax,[25] hemoperitoneum, or hemobilia[26] after liver biopsy. Relevant to this discussion, Gunawan and colleagues[17] clearly showed the relative safety of aminocaproic acid in patients who have liver disease.

THERAPEUTIC VERSUS PROPHYLACTIC THERAPY WITH PRO-COAGULANTS

A definite answer is not available regarding the issue of prophylaxis versus rescue therapy using these agents but rather can only indicate areas of uncertainty and the need for clinical research. Foremost is the need to better define the nature of the coagulopathy in a given patient who has liver disease at given time. Different strategies can be used optimally only when the true nature of the problem is fully revealed. Most clearly, INR and prothrombin time offer a very limited amount of information in this regard. Nonetheless, based on clinical experience and reasoning, rFVIIa and antifibrinolytics can be used to control hemorrhage and bleeding. For now, prophylactic administration is recommended in the most high-risk situations, such as using rFVIIa during intracranial pressure monitor placement when the occurrence of bleeding could lead quickly to irreversible injury with little or no opportunity for rescue intervention[27] (see article on fulminant liver failure by Munoz and colleagues elsewhere in this issue). However, because of the uncertain thrombotic risk and costs, prophylactic intervention in common procedures with these agents is probably not warranted and their use is best reserved as a rescue measure unless hyperfibrinolysis is already established or ongoing bleeding is present.

SUMMARY

This article reviews studies on the use of activated FVIIa and antifibrinolytics in patients who have liver disease. Many of the studies show some potential efficacy of these alternatives to traditional use of plasma. However, measuring the effect on bleeding risk is limited by the accuracy of the current conventional tests to assess coagulation (eg, INR, prothrombin time). Moreover, the potential benefits of these agents and other newer alternatives, such as prothrombin complexes, also must be balanced with the cost and an increase in thrombotic risk that couples their use. Considering these variables, the exact role of these agents has not been fully determined. Clinical investigation using more refined end points and patient stratification is needed to establish their role in the algorithm as a rescue or prophylactic agent and to investigate effective doses.

REFERENCES

1. Kessler CM. New products for managing inhibitors to coagulation factors: a focus on recombinant factor VIIa concentrate. Curr Opin Hematol 2000;7:408–13.
2. Hedner U, Glazer S, Pingel K, et al. Successful use of recombinant factor VIIa in patient with severe haemophilia a during synovectomy. Lancet 1988;2:1193.
3. Franchini M, Zaffanello M, Veneri D. Recombinant factor VIIa. An update on its clinical use. Thromb Haemost 2005;93:1027–35.

4. Bernstein DE, Jeffers L, Erhardtsen E, et al. Recombinant factor VIIa corrects prothrombin time in cirrhotic patients: a preliminary study. Gastroenterology 1997;113:1930–7.

5. Jeffers L, Chalasani N, Balart L, et al. Safety and efficacy of recombinant factor VIIa in patients with liver disease undergoing laparoscopic liver biopsy. Gastroenterology 2002;123:118–26.

6. Bosch J, Thabut D, Bendtsen F, et al. Recombinant factor VIIa for upper gastrointestinal bleeding in patients with cirrhosis: a randomized, double-blind trial. Gastroenterology 2004;127:1123–30.

7. Romero-Castro R, Jimenez-Saenz M, Pellicer-Bautista F, et al. Recombinant-activated factor VII as hemostatic therapy in eight cases of severe hemorrhage from esophageal varices. Clin Gastroenterol Hepatol 2004;2:78–84.

8. Bosch J, Thabut D, Albillos A, et al. Recombinant factor VIIa for variceal bleeding in patients with advanced cirrhosis: a randomized, controlled trial. Hepatology 2008;47:1604–14.

9. Shami VM, Caldwell SH, Hespenheide EE, et al. Recombinant activated factor VII for coagulopathy in fulminant hepatic failure compared with conventional therapy. Liver Transpl 2003;9:138–43.

10. Porte RJ, Caldwell SH. The role of recombinant factor VIIa in liver transplantation. Liver Transpl 2005;11:872–4.

11. Planinsic RM, van der Meer J, Testa G, et al. Safety and efficacy of a single bolus administration of recombinant factor VIIa in liver transplantation due to chronic liver disease. Liver Transpl 2005;11:895–900.

12. Lindley CM, Sawyer WT, Macik BG, et al. Pharmacokinetics and pharmacodynamics of recombinant factor VIIa. Clin Pharmacol Ther 1994;55:638–48.

13. Lodge JP, Jonas S, Jones RM, et al. Efficacy and safety of repeated perioperative doses of recombinant factor VIIa in liver transplantation. Liver Transpl 2005;11:973–9.

14. Moisescu E, Ardelean L, Simion I, et al. Recombinant factor VIIa treatment of bleeding associated with acute renal failure. Blood Coagul Fibrinolysis 2000;11:575–7.

15. Northup Pg HA, Caldwell SH. Factor VII versus FFP for bleeding associated with percutaneous liver biopsy: a cost-effectiveness evaluation. [Poster]. American Association for the Study of Liver Diseases, 57th Annual Meeting. Boston MA. Hepatology 2006;44:466A.

16. Mannucci PM. Hemostatic drugs. N Engl J Med 1998;339:245–53.

17. Gunawan B, Runyon B. The efficacy and safety of epsilon-aminocaproic acid treatment in patients with cirrhosis and hyperfibrinolysis. Aliment Pharmacol Ther 2006;23:115–20.

18. Royston D, Bidstrup BP, Taylor KM, et al. Effect of aprotinin on need for blood transfusion after repeat open-heart surgery. Lancet 1987;2:1289–91.

19. Xia VW, Steadman RH. Antifibrinolytics in orthotopic liver transplantation: current status and controversies. Liver Transpl 2005;11:10–8.

20. Porte RJ, Molenaar IQ, Begliomini B, et al. Aprotinin and transfusion requirements in orthotopic liver transplantation: a multicentre randomised double-blind study. EMSALT study group. Lancet 2000;355:1303–9.

21. Garcia-Huete L, Domenech P, Sabate A, et al. The prophylactic effect of aprotinin on intraoperative bleeding in liver transplantation: a randomized clinical study. Hepatology 1997;26:1143–8.

22. Dalmau A, Sabate A, Acosta F, et al. Tranexamic acid reduces red cell transfusion better than epsilon-aminocaproic acid or placebo in liver transplantation. Anesth Analg 2000;91:29–34.

23. Mannucci PM, Levi M. Prevention and treatment of major blood loss. N Engl J Med 2007;356:2301–11.
24. Djulbegovic B, Marasa M, Pesto A, et al. Safety and efficacy of purified factor IX concentrate and antifibrinolytic agents for dental extractions in hemophilia B. Am J Hematol 1996;51:168–70.
25. De Boer WA, Koolen MG, Roos CM, et al. Tranexamic acid treatment of hemothorax in two patients with malignant mesothelioma. Chest 1991;100:847–8.
26. Schwartz SI. Biliary tract surgery and cirrhosis: a critical combination. Surgery 1981;90:577–83.
27. Stravitz RT, Kramer AH, Davern T, et al. Intensive care of patients with acute liver failure: recommendations of the U.S. acute liver failure study group. Crit Care Med 2007;35:2498–508.

Coagulopathy of Acute Liver Failure

Santiago J. Munoz, MD, FACP, FACG[a,b,]*,
R. Todd Stravitz, MD, FACP, FACG[c],
Don A. Gabriel, MD, PhD[d]

KEYWORDS

- Coagulopathy • Liver • Hepatitis • Fulminant
- Plasma • Factor VII • Clotting

Acute liver failure (ALF) is a syndrome characterized by the development of hepatic encephalopathy and coagulopathy within 24 weeks of the onset of acute liver disease.[1] Coagulopathy is an essential component of the ALF syndrome and reflects the central role of liver function in hemostasis. Although the initial definitions of ALF did not include coagulopathy as a required element for the diagnosis, clinicians have long since been aware that ALF is consistently accompanied by coagulopathy of varying severity. Once standardization of the prothrombin time test result via the International Normalized Ratio (INR) became widely used to assess coagulopathy,[2] a prolonged INR greater than 1.5 was required for the diagnosis of ALF.[3] The clinical consequences of mild coagulopathy in ALF are generally of little concern. However, severe coagulopathy can be associated with bleeding and also can be a major obstacle to the performance of invasive procedures in patients with ALF. The severity of the coagulopathy is also a useful prognostic tool in ALF and a dynamic indicator of the hepatic function. This review focuses on the epidemiology, pathophysiology, presentation, evaluation, and management of coagulopathy in ALF.

FREQUENCY AND SEVERITY

The earliest series of patients with ALF described the presence of associated coagulopathy with a broad range of severity.[4–7] An important factor in the variability of these

[a] University of Pennsylvania, School of Medicine, 3400 Spruce Street, Philadelphia, PA 19104, USA
[b] PENN Presbyterian Medical Center, 38th and Market Streets, MOB 220, Philadelphia, PA 19104, USA
[c] Section of Hepatology, Hume-Lee Transplant Center, PO Box 980341, Virginia Commonwealth University, Richmond, VA 23298-0341, USA
[d] Division of Hematology/Oncology, University of North Carolina School of Medicine, Chapel Hill, North Carolina, NC 27599, USA
* Corresponding author. PENN Presbyterian Medical Center, 38th and Market Streets, MOB 220, Philadelphia, PA 19104.
E-mail address: Santiago.Munoz@uphs.upenn.edu (S.J. Munoz).

Clin Liver Dis 13 (2009) 95–107
doi:10.1016/j.cld.2008.10.001
1089-3261/08/$ – see front matter © 2009 Elsevier Inc. All rights reserved.

liver.theclinics.com

observations was related to the heterogeneous thromboplastin substrates used in the assays of the prothrombin time test.[2] When standardized by INR, it is possible to have a glimpse at comparing the frequency, severity, and other characteristics of the coagulopathy in ALF series reported from different areas of the world. The largest body of prospective data on the coagulopathy of ALF has been gathered by the US Acute Liver Failure Study Group.[8] In more than 1000 patients with ALF, the mean INR was 3.8 ± 4.0 (range: 1.5 to greater than 10.0). The majority of ALF patients (81%) presented coagulopathy of moderate severity (INR between 1.5 and 5.0). Fourteen percent had INR between 5.0 and 10.0, and 5% had very severe coagulopathy at admission, with INR greater than 10.0. The etiology of the ALF appeared to be related to the severity of the coagulopathy (**Fig. 1**).[8] The worst coagulopathy was observed in ALF caused by hepatitis B virus infection, acetaminophen overdose, Wilson's disease, and Budd-Chiari syndrome. The severe coagulopathy associated with the latter entity may seem paradoxical, because a hypercoagulable state is often the underlying cause of this syndrome. However, this situation likely reflects limitations of conventional tests such as INR in predicting a bleeding diathesis versus simply reflecting liver synthetic function. In contrast, ALF related to the acute fatty liver of pregnancy, and to some extent, ALF attributable to acute hepatitis A virus infection had the least severe coagulopathy as defined by conventional measures.[8] Thrombocytopenia was frequently observed in patients with ALF with nearly 40% demonstrating platelet counts below 90,000/mL at admission.[8]

PATHOPHYSIOLOGY

The mechanisms of coagulopathy in ALF are multifactorial and have been reviewed in detail elsewhere.[9,10] They include diminished synthesis of procoagulant factors, impaired anticoagulant and fibrinolytic systems, and defective function and number of platelets. In some patients a component of disseminated intravascular coagulation is present (see later in this article). Most coagulation factors are synthesized by the hepatocytes. Acute liver injury leads to an early and substantial reduction in clotting factors, particularly factors VII and V.[11] Reduced synthesis caused by severe acute liver cell injury in ALF, coupled with the short half-life of these coagulation factors (**Table 1**), promptly leads to depletion and rapid development of coagulopathy. The severity of the coagulopathy may be out of proportion to other manifestations of

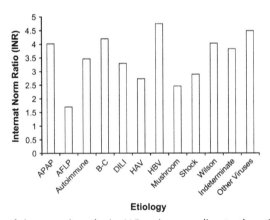

Fig. 1. The severity of the coagulopathy in ALF varies according to the etiology.

Table 1
Biological half-lives of liver-synthesized clotting factors

Clotting Factor	Half-Life
Fibrinogen	1.5–6.3 days
Prothrombin	2.8–4.4 days[a]
Factor V	12–36 hours
Factor VII	2–5 hours[a]
Factor IX	20–52 hours[a]
Factor X	32–48 hours[a]

[a] Vitamin K–dependent posttranslational carboxylation.

ALF. Thus, patients with profound encephalopathy (hepatic coma) may exhibit mild or moderate coagulopathy. Others with mild stage I-II hepatic encephalopathy may exhibit severe coagulopathy. The difference in clinical course between coagulopathy and encephalopathy was highlighted by a report that INR improved as ALF patients developed onset of hepatic encephalopathy in a recent study.[12]

CLINICAL PRESENTATION

The clinical significance of disordered coagulation in ALF requires consideration in two situations: spontaneous bleeding and iatrogenic bleeding after invasive procedures.

Spontaneous Bleeding

Although an abnormal prothrombin time test (INR) comprises part of the definition of ALF [1,3] and although its severity is related to prognosis,[13,14] spontaneous and clinically significant bleeding is rare in current experience (eg, ~5%).[15] However, earlier descriptive series of ALF suggested that spontaneous hemorrhage occurred frequently in ALF (50% to 70%).[16,17] It was severe in 30%,[18] and was the proximate cause of death in 27%.[19] The explanation for the apparent reduction in spontaneous bleeding in patients with ALF is unknown, but is unlikely due to the administration of prophylactic fresh frozen plasma.[19]

In contrast to patients with cirrhosis, bleeding in patients with ALF is generally "capillary-type" from mucosal lesions.[20,21] Whereas portal hypertension can accompany ALF because of the collapse of hepatic sinusoids,[21–23] bleeding from esophageal varices almost never occurs. Variceal bleeding in the setting of ALF should raise suspicion of Budd-Chiari syndrome. The most common site of bleeding in patients with ALF is from superficial gastric erosions.[15,19] To a lesser extent, it also presents spontaneously from nasopharyngeal, pulmonary, and genitourinary sources.[16,19,24] Suppression of gastric acid secretion with histamine-2 receptor antagonists (cimetidine) may decrease the risk of gastric mucosal bleeding, and thereby decrease transfusion requirements.[15,24] At present, proton pump inhibitors are more frequently used for prophylaxis against upper gastrointestinal bleeding in all patients with ALF.[25] This is in spite of the fact that gastric acid suppression has not been shown to improve survival.[15,24] Spontaneous intracranial bleeding has also been reported in patients with ALF, but is exceedingly rare (less than 1%) in the absence of insertion of an intracranial pressure (ICP) monitor.[14]

Iatrogenic Bleeding

Bleeding after invasive procedures constitutes a more significant problem in managing patients with ALF. Bleeding from venipuncture sites, seldom profuse,[20] may require prolonged tamponade. There are no data regarding the risk of significant bleeding after insertion of central venous catheters in patients with ALF. Some authorities consider the risk minor and advocate insertion after infusion of fresh frozen plasma without repeating the prothrombin time (Prof. J. Wendon, personal communication, 2007). The risk of intracranial bleeding after ICP monitor insertion remains one of the principal concerns regarding abnormal coagulation in ALF. In a large survey of ALF patients who underwent ICP monitor placement,[26] the risk of bleeding was proportional to the depth of insertion of the device. This was about 4%, 20%, and 22% in epidural, subdural, and parenchymal locations, respectively. In the same series, fatal hemorrhage occurred in 1%, 5%, and 4%. A more recent series documented intracranial hemorrhage in 10% of subjects, but half were incidental radiological findings, and bleeding may have contributed to the demise of the patient in only 3.5%.[27]

In selected patients with ALF, liver biopsy may improve diagnostic and prognostic accuracy, particularly in subjects with ALF of indeterminate etiology.[28,29] Transjugular liver biopsy has been performed with a low incidence of minor bleeding complications in patients with ALF. Even so, methods and target values to correct abnormal prothrombin times have not been detailed.[28,29]

Bleeding During and After Orthotopic Liver Transplantation (OLT)

Serious bleeding rarely complicates OLT for ALF despite profoundly abnormal parameters of coagulation preoperatively. As opposed to patients undergoing OLT for cirrhosis, patients with ALF generally have minimal portal hypertension (with the exception of ALF due to Budd-Chiari syndrome), no intra-abdominal varices, and do not have the peritoneal fibrosis that often complicates long-standing ascites, all of which lower the risk of bleeding complications. Preoperative parameters of coagulation (INR) do not predict intraoperative blood losses either in children[30] or adults undergoing OLT for ALF.[31] Even severe coagulopathy does not predict adverse outcomes after OLT (either at the time of admission or at the time of surgery).[32–35] Indeed, death from intra-abdominal hemorrhage after OLT has been reported in only 1% to 7% of patients transplanted for ALF.[33,34,36] However, high intraoperative transfusion requirements in patients undergoing OLT for ALF adversely affect graft and patient survival rates;[31,35] therefore, some transplant surgeons recommend correction of coagulation abnormalities throughout the procedure.[31]

LABORATORY EVALUATION

The following is a list of hemostatic parameters that may be helpful in the evaluation of bleeding risk and thrombosis in patients with ALF:

- Prothrombin time (INR)
- Platelet count and function (Assessment of platelet function in a timely and accurate manner remains a significant clinical problem.)
- Anti thrombin III level
- Indicators of fibrinolysis (D-dimer, plasmin(ogen), TAFI, PAI-1)
- Factor levels, especially FVIII, FV, FVII, and fibrinogen (Factors V and VII are also used as prognostic tools in acute liver failure. Low factor VIII in acute liver failure suggests disseminated intravascular coagulation.)
- Von Willebrand factor

- $_2$ Macroglobulin level
- Protein C and S levels

Although the source for hemostasis abnormalities in patients with ALF remains controversial, a vast literature exists documenting the importance of bleeding in patients with ALF.[9,21,36–40] Because the liver is the major site of synthesis of hemostatic factors including both procoagulant and anticoagulant factors, disease processes that adversely affect hepatocyte function can lead to an imbalance between procoagulant and anticoagulant pathways; bleeding often results.[5,41,42] ALF typically shows a more severe coagulation disturbance than cirrhosis.[5,41]

Most commonly, both procoagulant and anticoagulant factor levels are reduced producing a risk for hemorrhage and to a lesser extent, thrombosis. As a participant in this process, the liver's reticuloendothelial system normally removes activated procoagulants from circulation, thus providing a mechanism for the regulation of hemostasis. In ALF, the liver may not be able to perform this important function. Failure to remove activated procoagulants may also contribute to the development of a picture suggesting disseminated intravascular coagulation (DIC).[43] DIC may initially present as thrombosis, but later as a severe hemorrhagic diathesis.[44,45] Hemorrhage results because of both procoagulant factor depletion and from the presence of inhibitors.[44,45] Vascular ulcerations and thrombocytopenia enhance the risk of bleeding in this syndrome.

Distinguishing DIC from fibrinolysis may be difficult especially since some degree of fibrinolysis often accompanies DIC as evidenced by the presence of fibrin split products. End-organ microthrombi, if present, suggest DIC while normal ATIII, normal Factor VIII, and absence of microthrombi suggests predominant fibrinolysis. When present, DIC may initially present as thrombosis, but later as a severe hemorrhagic diathesis.[44,45] However, in many clinical situations the picture is mixed in a condition that some have called AICF (Accelerated Intravascular Coagulation and Fibrinolysis). This term is itself misleading and a more accurate term would include "accelerated thrombin production," which reflects the potentially important role of coexisting variables such as infection on thrombin production. Clearly, the field is one that is very promising for productive clinical-laboratory research. In this regard, assays to better characterize this complicated picture, including accelerated thrombin production, are currently under development.

A hallmark of ALF is depressed synthesis of most procoagulants. This is especially true of FII, FV, FVII, and FX, with the exception of FVIII, which is often elevated.[9,38,46] Factor depression can result from decreased production, increased consumption, or both. As with cirrhosis, dysfibrinogenemias may also occur in ALF,[47–50] and be manifested as a fibrin assembly abnormality. Cryoglobulins occur in some patients with hepatitis C. Among other problems, it may also cause fibrin assembly anomalies.

Assessment of factor deficiency in liver disease is most often based on the prothrombin time (PT) and activated partial thromboplastin time (aPTT). Recent evidence indicates that the very high INR values typically observed in ALF are often misleading as an indicator of the severity of liver disease (see also the article by Tripodi in this issue).[10,51] The PT was developed to monitor warfarin therapy, in which INR values are lower than those in ALF. There are problems associated with the use of the PT to evaluate coagulopathy in ALF. For example, it does not assess anticoagulation factors or cellular contributions such as platelets to hemostasis[10] Another major problem with the PT and its associated INR arises from differences in the sensitivity of the thromboplastin reagents used in the PT assay.[52,53] Regression lines comparing various thromboplastins in ALF show a different slope when compared with patients anticoagulated with warfarin.[53]

Another common complication of ALF is activation of the fibrinolytic system,[54] particularly in association with liver transplant (see also the article by Ferro and colleagues in this issue). Because the PT and aPTT do not correlate with hyperfibrinolysis, other diagnostic tests are needed. Hyperfibrinolysis in ALF is related to decreased clearance of plasminogen activators in the liver.[55,56] Fibrinolysis elevates plasma levels of fibrin degradation products. These subsequently inhibit activated procoagulants, especially fibrin assembly and thrombin. Fibrin degradation products may also bind the fibrinogen receptor, integrin $\alpha_{IIb}\beta_3$, on the platelet surface. It may similarly inhibit platelet aggregation that can cause bleeding.

Plasma levels of another anticoagulant molecule, antithrombin III, are typically low in ALF, while the thrombin-antithrombin complex (TAT) is elevated. Kerr and colleagues[38] reviewed 663 patients with liver disease compared with 547 healthy subjects. They showed that depression of both antithrombin III level and plasminogen indicate a poor patient survival.[38] In another clinical study, Boyadjian[57] showed that depressed plasminogen levels and an elevated antithrombin III level suggested clinical improvement. Boks and colleagues[20] reviewed hemorrhagic outcomes in patients with hepatic failure. In this study, three groups including ALF were assessed. Depression of procoagulants, antithrombin III, plasminogen, and α2antiplasmin, as well as prekallikrein, were significantly lower in ALF.[20]

Yamaguchi and colleagues[42] have shown that decreased activation of protein C occurs in severe liver failure along with endothelial cell damage. The anti-inflammatory role of activated protein C (APC) and its effect on cytokine production in severe liver disease were also examined.[42] Elevated levels of tumor necrosis factor (TNF)-α were found to correlate with low levels of protein C. Although levels of thrombin activable fibrinolysis inhibitors (TAFI) are depressed in cirrhosis, an increase in bleeding does not occur as a result of the depressed TAFI levels.[58]

Both the platelet count and platelet function can be adversely affected by ALF. Thrombocytopenia may result from decreased platelet production, increased destruction, or sequestration. In cirrhosis, thrombocytopenia is common. It is often associated with portal hypertension and with decreased thrombopoietin (TPO) production.[10] Conversely, in acute hepatitis, TPO is usually elevated and does not correlate with the platelet count.[59,60] In fulminant hepatitis, TPO levels may actually be depressed.[59] An autoimmune mechanism for thrombocytopenia in ALF has also been proposed.[61,62]

A wide variety of platelet function abnormalities has been reported. Decreased platelet activation in response to common agonists such as ADP, thrombin, thromboxane A2, and collagen platelet adhesion has been observed.[63,64] Abnormalities in platelet adhesion under flow conditions have been found.[65] von Willebrand factor may play a role in the defective platelet adhesion.[36]

MANAGEMENT

Strategies for management of coagulopathy of ALF include the following: monitoring and observation, prophylaxis in the absence of bleeding, preemptive therapy before invasive procedures, and coagulopathy therapy associated with active bleeding. The main therapeutic tools include replacement of clotting factors via administration of fresh frozen plasma (FFP), cryoprecipitate, recombinant activated factor VII (rFVIIa), exchange plasmapheresis, platelets concentrates, combinations of the above, and vitamin K.

Prophylactic administration of FFP or other hemostatic factors to simply correct the prothrombin time is not justified in ALF. Such a practice obscures the value of the prothrombin time as a dynamic indicator of recovering or worsening liver function, and may also lead to fluid overload or TRALI (see also the articles by Shah and Argo in this issue). An older study in which FFP was administered to patients with ALF and coagulopathy demonstrated no benefit on outcome.[18] Whether prophylaxis with FFP is useful in nonbleeding patients with very severe coagulopathy (INR > 7.0) is unknown; however, patients with very severe coagulopathy often exhibit mucosal or venopuncture sites bleeding. This frequently leads clinicians to initiate therapy with FFP. If the patient with ALF develops overt bleeding (mucosal, gastrointestinal, genitourinary, hematomas), there is a clinical rationale to treat the coagulopathy. This also applies to severe thrombocytopenia if present, as well as to the mechanical measures to control the bleeding complication.

An attempt to partially correct the coagulopathy is often necessary in preparation for an invasive procedure. Patients with ALF may require procedures such as transjugular or percutaneous liver biopsy, placement of an intracranial pressure transducer, paracentesis or thoracentesis, and of course, some will undergo urgent liver transplantation. In these instances, the operator performing the procedure will often request correction of the coagulopathy, typically but not always, to an INR value equal or below 1.5. It should be noted that there is no evidence-based data indicating that therapy of the coagulopathy is beneficial (ie, leading to decreased bleeding risk with the invasive procedure). Similarly, there are no adequate data on the extent to which the coagulopathy should be corrected.

Nonetheless (since the request to correct the coagulopathy before an invasive procedure remains a widespread practice), some approaches to accomplish the correction are discussed later in this article. Similar strategies are also used to treat coagulopathy in the setting of active bleeding. Administration of FFP is the most common treatment modality used to treat the coagulopathy of ALF.[7,8] In a recent large series, patients with ALF received an average of 13.7 ± 15.0 units of FFP during the first week of admission.[8] The overall efficacy of FFP to correct the INR, a clinical broadly used surrogate marker of coagulopathy, is moderate. Furthermore, the effect of FFP on the INR demonstrates considerable variability among patients. With FFP alone, very severe coagulopathy rarely corrects to the INR range where operators feel comfortable performing invasive procedures in ALF (INR of approximately 1.5). DIC should be suspected when administration of FFP causes little or no improvement in a markedly prolonged INR.

The major limitation of FFP when used to correct coagulopathy in ALF is the high potential to cause volume overload and associated consequences or hypersensitivity reactions. As a result, the use of activated recombinant factor VII (rFVIIa) has been explored in ALF.[66,67] Shami and colleagues[66] reported dramatic improvement in INR with relatively modest doses of rFVIIa (**Fig. 2**). Quan and colleagues[67] investigated the possibility that sequential or combination therapy of FFP and rFVIIa could be more useful in the coagulopathy of ALF. In this preliminary report, rFVIIa at doses of 40 to 80 μg/kg in combination with FFP appeared more potent that rFVIIa alone.[67] Despite this, several important questions remain concerning the combined use of rFVIIa and FFP in ALF, including dosing schedule and the potential risk for thrombotic complications.[66–69]

More work is necessary to determine the optimal manner to use rFVIIa for the coagulopathy of ALF. Nonetheless, in cases of severe coagulopathy and clinically significant bleeding, or before invasive procedures, rFVIIa should be kept in mind as a useful therapeutic resource. Exchange plasmapheresis (EP) allows the transfusion of large amounts of FFP to patients with ALF.[70] The EP procedure involves an isovolumetric removal and transfusion of fresh plasma. This reduces the risk of volume overload

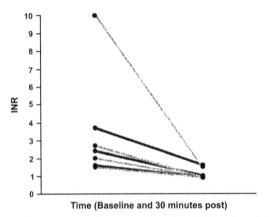

Fig. 2. PT INR before and 30 minutes after administration of 40 μg/kg of rFVIIa. (*From* Shami V, Caldwell S, Hespenheide E. Recombinant activated factor VII for coagulopathy of fulminant hepatic failure compared with conventional therapy. Liver Transplant 2003;9:138–43; with permission.)

while effectively correcting the INR (**Table 2**). EP is used extensively in Asian countries as a component of the standard management of ALF, but it is rarely used in Western areas for this purpose.[71–73]

There are even less data on which evidence-based recommendations can be issued for platelet transfusions in the setting of ALF. As with FFP, platelet replacement is not indicated in the absence of active bleeding. In the small number of ALF patients who exhibit extreme thrombocytopenia (<10,000/mL),[8] a hematological evaluation is necessary before simply administering platelet transfusions. Prophylactic platelet transfusion for ALF patients with platelet count between 10,000 and 30,000/mL is debatable. Given the universal coexistence of coagulopathy, extrapolation of bleeding risk from situations of severe thrombocytopenia without coagulopathy is probably inappropriate.

Fibrinogen is a key clotting factor synthesized by liver cells. Severe hypofibrinogenemia (level below 100 mg/dL) in the presence of active bleeding should be treated with administration of cryoprecipitate.[25] A notably decreased fibrinogen level may also reflect DIC. There is very little data on the clinical value of treating DIC and hyperfibrinolysis in the setting of ALF. An older study found no effect of heparin infusion on outcome in ALF, and bleeding occurred in about 25% of patients.[74] No evidence-based guidelines exist at this time for use of agents acting on fibrinolytic and anticoagulant systems in ALF because of the paucity of data. Last, vitamin K (10 mg

Table 2							
Effect of plasmapheresis on prothrombin time in acute liver failure							
	PT (sec)	INR	PTT (sec)	Fib mg/dL	Factor II (%)	Factor V (%)	Factor VII (%)	Factor IX (%)
Before	25.1	4.0	57	138	27	24	0	25
After	14.9	1.4	44	174	54	47	36	46

Abbreviations: Fib, fibrinogen; INR, International Normalized Ratio; PT, prothrombin time; PTT, partial thromboplastin time.

From Singer A, Olthoff K, Kim H, et al. Role of plasmapheresis in the management of acute hepatic failure in children. Ann Surg 2001;234:418–24; with permission.

subcutaneously daily for 3 days) should be given to all patients diagnosed with ALF to ensure that vitamin K deficiency is not a contributing factor to the coagulopathy.[75,76]

SUMMARY

Every patient with ALF develops coagulopathy, although this may or may not be associated with a net bleeding diathesis. The severity of the coagulopathy is moderate in most patients and its pathogenesis is multifactorial. Other hemostatic disorders found in these patients may include thrombocytopenia, DIC, and fibrinolysis. In spite of the coagulopathy, spontaneous bleeding in ALF is uncommon. The evaluation of the coagulopathy is most often based on the prothrombin time but this approach has several limitations. Management of the coagulopathy with transfusions of FFP is indicated only in the presence of active bleeding or before invasive procedures, especially with depressed fibrinogen levels. Correction of the coagulopathy is particularly important before liver biopsy or placement of an intracranial pressure transducer because of the potentially severe result of intracranial hemorrhage. The role of activated recombinant factor VII appears as a promising therapy for severe coagulopathy in ALF, but further evaluation is necessary before broad use of this clotting factor in this setting.

REFERENCES

1. Schiodt F, Atillasoy E, Shakil O, et al. Etiology and outcome for 295 patients with acute liver failure in the United States. Liver Transpl 1999;5:29–34.
2. Munoz S. Prothrombin time in fulminant hepatic failure. Gastroenterology 1991; 100:1480–9.
3. Ostapowicz G, Fontana R, Schiedt F, et al. Results of a prospective study of acute liver failure at 17 tertiary care centers in the United States. Ann Intern Med 2002; 137:947–54.
4. Trey C, Davidson CS. The management of fulminant hepatic failure. Prog Liver Dis 1970;3:282–98.
5. O'Grady JG, Langley PG, Isola L, et al. Coagulopathy of fulminant hepatic failure. Semin Liver Dis 1986;6(2):159–63.
6. Muñoz SJ. Difficult management problems in fulminant hepatic failure. Semin Liver Dis 1993;13(4):395–413.
7. Anand A, Nightingale P, Neuberger J. Early indicators of prognosis in fulminant hepatic failure: an assessment of the King's criteria. J Hepatol 1997;26:62–8.
8. Munoz S, Reddy R, Lee W, et al. Coagulopathy in acute liver failure. Neurocrit Care 2008;9:103–7.
9. Pereira SP, Langley PG, Williams R. The management of abnormalities of hemostasis in acute liver failure. Semin Liver Dis 1996;16:403–14.
10. Trotter JF. Coagulation abnormalities in patients who have liver disease. Clin Liver Dis 2006;10:665–78.
11. Cornillon B, Paul J, Belleville J, et al. Experimental DMNA induced hepatic necrosis: early course of haemostatic disorders in the rat. Comp Biochem Physiol 1985; 80:277–84.
12. Schmidt LE, Larsen FS. MELD score as a predictor of liver failure and death in patients with acetaminophen-induced liver injury. Hepatology 2007;45:789–96.
13. O'Grady JG, Alexander GJ, Hayllar KM, et al. Early indicators of prognosis in fulminant hepatic failure. Gastroenterology 1989;97:439–45.
14. Bernuau J, Benhamou JP. Fulminant and subfulminant liver failure. In: Bircher J, Benhamou JP, McIntyre N, editors. Oxford textbook of clinical hepatology. 2nd edition. Oxford (U.K.): Oxford University Press; 1999. p. 1341.

15. Macdougall BR, Bailey RJ, Williams R. H2-receptor antagonists and antacids in the prevention of acute gastrointestinal haemorrhage in fulminant hepatic failure. Two controlled trials. Lancet 1977;1:617–9.

16. Sherlock S. Fulminant hepatic failure. Adv Intern Med 1993;38:245–67.

17. Clark R, Rake MO, Flute PT, et al. Coagulation abnormalities in acute liver failure: pathogenetic and therapeutic implications. Scand J Gastroenterol Suppl 1973; 19:63–70.

18. Gazzard BG, Henderson JM, Williams R. Early changes in coagulation following a paracetamol overdose and a controlled trial of fresh frozen plasma therapy. Gut 1975;16:617–20.

19. Gazzard BG, Portmann B, Murray-Lyon IM, et al. Causes of death in fulminant hepatic failure and relationship to quantitative histological assessment of parenchymal damage. QJM 1975;44:615–26.

20. Boks AL, Brommer EJ, Schalm SW, et al. Hemostasis and fibrinolysis in severe liver failure and their relation to hemorrhage. Hepatology 1986;6:79–86.

21. Lisman T, Leebeek FW. Hemostatic alterations in liver disease: a review on pathophysiology, clinical consequences, and treatment. Dig Surg 2007;24(4): 250–8.

22. Valla D, Flejou JF, Lebrec D, et al. Portal hypertension and ascites in acute hepatitis: clinical, hemodynamic and histological correlations. Hepatology 1989;10: 482–7.

23. Lebrec D, Nouel O, Bernuau J, et al. Portal hypertension in fulminant viral hepatitis. Gut 1980;21:962–4.

24. Macdougall BR, Williams R. H2-receptor antagonist in the prevention of acute upper gastrointestinal hemorrhage in fulminant hepatic failure: a controlled trial. Gastroenterology 1978;74(2 Pt 2):464–5.

25. Stravitz RT, Kramer AH, Davern T, et al. Intensive care of patients with acute liver failure: recommendations of the U.S. Acute Liver Failure Study Group. Crit Care Med 2007;35(11):2498–508.

26. Blei AT, Olafsson S, Webster S, et al. Complications of intracranial pressure monitoring in fulminant hepatic failure. Lancet 1993;16(341):157–8.

27. Vaquero J, Fontana RJ, Larson AM, et al. Complications and use of intracranial pressure monitoring in patients with acute liver failure and severe encephalopathy. Liver Transpl 2005;11:1581–9.

28. Donaldson BW, Gopinath R, Wanless IR, et al. The role of transjugular liver biopsy in fulminant liver failure: relation to other prognostic indicators. Hepatology 1993; 18:1370–6.

29. Hanau C, Munoz S, Rubin R. Histopathological heterogeneity in fulminant hepatic failure. Hepatology 1995;21:345–51.

30. Carlier M, Van Obbergh LJ, Veyckemans F, et al. Hemostasis in children undergoing liver transplantation. Semin Thromb Hemost 1993;19(3):218–22.

31. Mor E, Jennings L, Gonwa TA, et al. The impact of operative bleeding on outcome in transplantation of the liver. Surg Gynecol Obstet 1993;176:219–27.

32. O'Grady JG, Alexander GJ, Thick M, et al. Outcome of orthotopic liver transplantation in the aetiological and clinical variants of acute liver failure. Q J Med 1988; 68:817–24.

33. Bernal W, Wendon J, Rela M, et al. Use and outcome of liver transplantation in acetaminophen-induced acute liver failure. Hepatology 1998;27:1050–5.

34. Devlin J, Wendon J, Heaton N, et al. Pretransplantation clinical status and outcome of emergency transplantation for acute liver failure. Hepatology 1995;21: 1018–24.

35. Farmer DG, Anselmo DM, Ghobrial RM, et al. Liver transplantation for fulminant hepatic failure: experience with more than 200 patients over a 17-year period. Ann Surg 2003;237:666–75.
36. Lisman T, Leebeek FWG, de Groot PG. Haemostatic abnormalities in patients with liver disease. J Hepatol 2002;37:280–7.
37. Lentschener C, Roche K, Ozier Y. A review of aprotinin in orthotopic liver transplantation: can its harmful effects offset its beneficial effects? Anesth Analg 2005;100:1248–55.
38. Kerr R, Newsome P, Germain L, et al. Effects of acute liver injury on blood coagulation. J Thromb Haemost 2003;1:754–9.
39. Hughes RD, Nicolaou N, Langley PG, et al. Plasma cytokine levels and coagulation and complement activation during use of the extracorporeal liver assist device in acute liver failure. Artif Organs 1998;22:854–8.
40. Scherer R, Gille A, Erhard J, et al. The effect of substitution with AT II- and PPSB-concentrates in patients with terminal lover insufficiency. Anaesthesist 1994;43:178–82.
41. Langley PG, Forbes A, Hughes RD, et al. Thrombin-antithrombin III complex in fulminate hepatic failure: evidence for disseminated intravascular coagulation and relationship to outcome. Eur J Clin Invest 1990;20:627–31.
42. Yamaguchi M, Gabazza EC, Taguchi O, et al. Decreased protein C in patients with fulminant hepatic failure. Scand J Gastroenterol 2006;41:331–7.
43. Ben-Ari Z, Osman E, Hutton RA, et al. Disseminated intravascular coagulation in liver cirrhosis: fact or fiction? Am J Gastroenterol 1999;94:2977–82.
44. Hirata K, Ohata Y, Fujiwara K. Hepatic sinusoidal cell destruction in the development of intravascular coagulation in acute liver failure of rats. J Pathol 1989;158:157–65.
45. Mochida S, Arai M, Ohno A, et al. Deranged blood coagulation equilibrium as a factor of massive liver necrosis following endotoxin administration in partially hepatectomized rats. Hepatology 1999;29:1532–40.
46. Langley PG, Hughes RD, Williams R. Increased factor VIII complex in fulminant hepatic failure. Thromb Haemost 1985;54:693–6.
47. Kelly DA, Summerfield JA. Hemostasis in liver disease. Semin Liver Dis 1987;7:182–91.
48. Francis JL. Acquired dysfibrinogenemia in liver disease. J Clin Pathol 1982;35:667–72.
49. Green G, Thomson JM, Dymock IW, et al. Abnormal fibrin polymerization in liver disease. Br J Haematol 1976;34:427–39.
50. Carr ME, Gabriel DA. Altered plasma viscosity and shear dependent gelation of an IgM cryoglobulin. Clin Hemorheol 1987;6:529–40.
51. Tripodi A, Salerno F, Chantarangkul V, et al. Evidence of normal thrombin generation in cirrhosis despite abnormal conventional coagulation tests. Hepatology 2005;41:553–8.
52. Robert A, Chazouilleres O. Prothrombin time in liver failure: time, ratio, activity percentage, or international normalized ratio? Hepatology 1996;24:1392–4, Ewe K.Dig Dis Dci 1981;26:973–93.
53. Dillon JF, Simpson JK, Hayes PC. Liver biopsy bleeding time: an unpredictable event. J Gastroenterol Hepatol 1994;9:269–71.
54. Caldwell SH, Hoffman M, Lisman T, et al. Coagulation disorders and hemostasis in liver disease: pathology and critical assessment of current management. Hepatology 2006;44:1039–46.

55. Rappaport S. Coagulation problems in liver disease. Blood Coagul Fibrinolysis 2000;11(Suppl 1):S69–74.
56. Amitrano L, Guardascione MA, Brancaccio V, et al. Coagulation disorders in liver disease. Semin Liver Dis 2002;22:83–96.
57. Boyadjian HP. Prognostic significance of antithrombin III, plasminogen and pro-activatios of plasminogen activity in viral hepatitis. Dtsch Z Verdau Stoffwechselkr 1988;48:83–93.
58. Lisman T, Leebeek FW, Mosier LO, et al. Thrombin-activatable fibrinolysis inhibitor deficiency in cirrhosis is not associated with increased fibrinolysis. Gastroenterology 2001;121:131–9.
59. Okumoto K, Siato T, Onodera M, et al. Serum levels of stem cell factor and thrombopoietin are markedly decreased in fulminant hepatic failure patients with a poor prognosis. J Gastroenterol Hepatol 2007;8:1171–3.
60. Schiodt FV, Balko J, Schilsky ME, et al. Thrombopoietin in acute liver failure. Hepatology 2003;37:558–61.
61. Pereira J, Accatino L, Alfaro J, et al. Platelet autoantibodies in patients with chronic liver disease. Am J Hematol 1995;50:173–8.
62. Pockros PJ, Duchini A, McMillan R, et al. Immune thrombocytopenic purpura in patients with chronic hepatitis C virus infection. Am J Gastroenterol 2002;97: 2040–5.
63. Escolar G, Cases A, Vinas M, et al. Evaluation of acquired platelet dysfunction in uremic and cirrhotic patients using the platelet analyzed PFQ100: influence of hematocrit elevation. Haematologica 1999;84:614–9.
64. Laffi G, Cominelli F, Ruggiero M, et al. Altered platelet function in cirrhosis of the liver: impairment of inositol lipid and arachidonic acid metabolism in response to agonists. epatHhHH. Hepatology 1988;8:1620–6.
65. Ordinas A, Escolar G, Cirera, et al. Defective signal transduction in platelets from cirrhosis is associated with increased cyclic nucleotides. Gastroenterology 1993; 105:148–56.
66. Shami V, Caldwell S, Hespenheide E. Recombinant activated factor VII for coagulopathy of fulminant hepatic failure compared with conventional therapy. Liver Transpl 2003;9:138–43.
67. Quan D, Bass N, Hirose R, et al. The effect of recombinant factor VIIa and fresh frozen plasma on the INR in patients with acute and chronic liver failure. Hepatology 2003;38(4):550A.
68. Porte R, Caldwell S. The role of recombinant factor VIIa in liver transplantation. Liver Transpl 2005;11:872–4.
69. Pavese P, Bonadona A, Beaubien J, et al. FVIIa corrects the coagulopathy of liver failure but may be associated with thrombosis: a report of four cases. Can J Anaesth 2005;52:26–9.
70. Munoz S, Ballas S, Moritz M, et al. Perioperative management of fulminant and subfulminant liver failure with therapeutic plasmapheresis. Transplant Proc 1989;21:3535–6.
71. Takahashi T, Malchesky P, Nose Y. Artificial liver: state of the art. Dig Dis Sci 1991; 36:1327–40.
72. Akamatsu K, Tanaka Y, Tada K, et al. Filtration of fresh frozen plasma used as substitution fluid in plasma exchange in order to remove microaggregates. Artif Organs 1990;14:429–35.
73. Takahashi Y, Shimizu M. Aetiology and prognosis of fulminant viral hepatitis in Japan: a multicentre study. J Gastroenterol Hepatol 1991;6:159–64.

74. Gazzard B, Clark R, Borirakchanyavat V, et al. A controlled trial of heparin therapy in the coagulation defect of paracetamol-induced hepatic necrosis. Gut 1974;15: 89–93.
75. Pereira S, Rowbotham D, Fitt S, et al. Pharmacokinetics and efficacy of oral versus intravenous mixed-micellar phylloquinone (vitamin K1) in severe acute liver disease. J Hepatol 2005;42:365–70.
76. Reverter JC. Abnormal hemostasis tests and bleeding in chronic liver disease: are they related? Yes. J Thromb Haemost 2006;4:717–20.

Hypercoagulation in Liver Disease

Patrick G. Northup, MD, MHS

KEYWORDS

- Cirrhosis • Hypercoagulation • Thrombophilia
- Coagulation disorders • Venous thromboembolism
- Pulmonary embolism • Portopulmonary hypertension

Hypercoagulation or thrombophilia refers to the propensity for inappropriate clot formation. Although bleeding is the most commonly recognized clinical concern in patients who have chronic liver disease and cirrhosis, increasing evidence also shows that inappropriate clot formation plays a key role in the coagulation disorders of chronic liver disease. This article provides a brief overview of the modern understanding of the endogenous anticoagulant system and some of the known and suspected disruptions of this system in cirrhosis. The possible consequences of a hypercoagulation syndrome in patients who have liver disease are reviewed and the implications for future research areas and treatment modalities are assessed in this and two other articles in this issue (by Anstee and colleagues and Bittencourt and colleagues, respectively).

The coagulation system is a complex balance of procoagulant and anticoagulant components that function in a unique homeostasis and provide a rapid response to endothelial disruption with fibrin deposition, platelet aggregation, and clot formation (see also the articles by Monroe and Hoffman elsewhere in this issue). In the healthy state, this coagulation response is elegantly balanced by an anticoagulation response that prevents inappropriate clot extension, minimizes local ischemia, and promotes eventual clot breakdown once hemostasis is secured. In the diseased state an imbalance may lead to domination of one side of the coagulation equation: some patients may experience excessive bleeding, whereas others may experience excessive clotting. The side of the equation that becomes dominant in any specific patient is not easily predictable.

The liver is the primary site for production of many of the procoagulant clotting factors, namely factors II, V, VII, IX, X, and XI. Relative deficiencies in these factors may be primarily responsible for increased bleeding tendency. Conversely, evidence shows that decreased production of endogenous anticoagulants, such as protein C, protein S, thrombomodulin, and tissue plasminogen activator (t-PA), may lead to an imbalance favoring clotting in some patients (see also the article by Tripodi in this

Division of Gastroenterology and Hepatology, University of Virginia Health System, JPA and Lee Streets, MSB 2142, Charlottesville VA 22908–0708, USA
E-mail address: pgn5qs@virginia.edu

Clin Liver Dis 13 (2009) 109–116
doi:10.1016/j.cld.2008.09.003
1089-3261/08/$ – see front matter © 2009 Elsevier Inc. All rights reserved.

liver.theclinics.com

volume).[1,2] This imbalance is further complicated by the fact that patients who have cirrhosis have a generalized decrease in protein production, which results in a limited quantitative reserve of factors on either side of the coagulation equation. These patients therefore have an inability to compensate for even mild fluctuations in local environments that might otherwise be effectively buffered in healthy patients who have a larger functional reserve. Review of the known endogenous procoagulant systems and their alteration in patients who have cirrhosis will help in understanding the consequences of hypercoagulation.

LIVER DISEASE AND THE COAGULATION SYSTEM

The advent of aggressive therapeutic anticoagulation for various clinical disorders over the past decades has expanded the knowledge of the innate procoagulant system. Fundamentally, hemostasis is composed of four basic building blocks: vasoconstriction, the platelet, the traditional extrinsic and intrinsic clotting factors along with the thrombin burst, and finally the fibrin mesh. Although this concept is a significant oversimplification, this discussion focuses on each of these underlying building blocks and their derangements in liver disease.

The immediate response to vascular injury is autonomic vasoconstriction, which is potentiated or antagonized by numerous locally and systemically active mediators, including nitric oxide,[3,4] the eicosanoids,[5,6] endothelin,[7] and the ecto-nucleotidases (ADPase/CD39).[8] These agents are early mediators in the clotting process and their actions may promote vascular reactions depending on their local concentration at the site of the injury. This fact underscores the difficulty in any global assay of coagulation, because local conditions near the site of injury may vary remarkably from systemic conditions. This variability is present especially in the pathophysiology of cirrhosis, which is characterized by systemic vasodilation and the resulting vascular stasis. This stasis is also evident on the splanchnic side of the circulation and may lead to inappropriately high local levels of vasoactive agents or procoagulation factors and may contribute to the high prevalence of portal vein thrombosis in cirrhosis patients.[9] Liver disease has been shown to affect the levels of nitric oxide and the endothelins, and fluctuations in these levels have been linked to the complications of liver disease, such as systemic hypotension[10] and the hepatorenal syndrome.[11]

Platelets are a key component of the early clotting mechanism. After tissue injury, the initial exposure of tissue factor to the local environment eventually produces a thrombin burst that activates platelets through an association of the von Willebrand factor (vWF) and factor VIII (fVIII). Through a positive feedback loop fundamentally based on more thrombin production, more platelets are recruited and activated to establish the platelet plug. This plug is initially unstable until the fibrin mesh is crosslinked to form a more mature clot. The regulation and breakdown of the platelet plug is poorly understood, but vWF levels influence the ability of platelets to adhere to each other. Local disassociation of vWF with fVIII likely leads to platelet disaggregation. Thrombocytopenia is a hallmark of cirrhosis, which may also be associated with platelet dysfunction. Despite this fact, highly elevated levels of vWF have been shown in cirrhosis[12] and local persistence of vWF could be associated with increased platelet aggregability.

Regulatory throttling of the clotting factor cascade is primarily effected through the protein C pathway. The thrombin-burst positive feedback loop produces large amounts of thrombin from inactive prothrombin and serves as priming for the clotting cascade. Early in the clot formation process, thrombin acts as procoagulant through amplification of factor V and VIII, recruitment of activated platelets, and conversion of fibrinogen to fibrin. However, as hemostasis is achieved, thrombin is cleaved by anti-thrombin (through the action of antithrombin III) and active thrombin concentrations drop.

Thrombin is also bound to thrombomodulin and this complex activates protein C (aPC), which is the major negative feedback mechanism serving to limit clot extension. Protein S is a critical nonenzymatic cofactor in the clot moderation cascade and is required for the function of aPC. The aPC/protein S complex converts Va and VIIIa to inactive compounds and restrains the clotting process. Congenital genetic defects in protein C, protein S, antithrombin III, and prothrombin production are well-known causes of inappropriate thrombosis.

It has been documented that in patients with cirrhosis, serum levels of all of these proteins can be low because of decreased production.[1,2] The procoagulant factors prothrombin, V, VII, IX, X, and XI[13] are also commonly low in patients who have liver disease. Despite these relative factor deficiencies, thrombin production is normal in cirrhosis.[14] Therefore, with the depleted reserves in chronic liver disease, a small fluctuation resulting in local protein C deficiency might lead to a prothrombotic environment and favor clot formation in some settings.

Finally, the immature platelet plug is restrained and solidified with a fibrin polymer mesh to form the final mature clot. Once hemostasis and endothelial healing is achieved, the fibrin mesh is degraded by the serine protease plasmin. Inactive plasminogen is activated to plasmin through the actions of t-PA and urokinase plasminogen activator (u-PA). The unfortunately named plasminogen activator inhibitor 1 serves to moderate this activation and therefore promote clot stability. Similarly, α_2 plasmin inhibitor directly inactivates plasmin, also promoting clot stability. Although studies of this system in patients who have cirrhosis have been sparse, some investigators have found a relative persistence of t-PA and u-PA.[15,16] This effect is often ambiguously described as low-grade disseminated intravascular coagulation and is potentiated by endotoxemia.[17] A shortened euglobulin lysis time, which is typical of hyperfibrinolysis, is seen in 31% of hospitalized patients who have cirrhosis.[18] However, the typical syndrome of disseminated intravascular coagulation with fibrin deposition in the tissues[19] and mucosal bleeding is much less common in all but the most critically ill patients who have cirrhosis.

Consequences of Hypercoagulation in Cirrhosis

Macrovascular thrombotic disease

The basic pathophysiology of the coagulation system in patients who have cirrhosis lays the groundwork for circumstances that can lead to a hypercoagulable state in these patients. The clinical expression of this syndrome is often unrecognized by practitioners who may be focused on the bleeding risk in cirrhosis and the conventional laboratory tests of coagulation parameters that complicate the everyday medical care in these patients. A hypercoagulation syndrome in patients who have cirrhosis may manifest itself as macrovascular thrombosis, such as portal vein thrombosis, deep (nonsplanchnic) venous thrombosis (DVT), and pulmonary embolism (PE). However, accumulating data also implicate microvascular thrombosis in nonhepatic end-organ damage and more insidiously in progression of cirrhosis to atrophy (see article by Anstee and colleagues elsewhere in this issue).

The prevalence of extrahepatic portal vein thrombosis (PVT) in patients who have cirrhosis ranges from 2.95% to 13.8%[20,21] (see article by Bittencourt and colleagues elsewhere in this issue). In patients who have hepatocellular carcinoma or previous surgical portosystemic shunt placement, the prevalence is as high as 34.8%.[20] Because many of the thromboses occur in patients who have decompensated Child's

C cirrhosis, the symptoms of a PVT, such as worsening of ascites or precipitation of an esophageal variceal bleeding event, may be attributed to worsening of cirrhosis without recognition of underlying PVT unless imaging studies are performed. Thus, the ability to clearly define incidence rates is limited.

The origin of a PVT is clearly multifactorial in most patients who have cirrhosis, and these thromboses are usually attributed to a combination of the low flow state in the obstructed portal vein, malignant invasion, and, less commonly, to systemic hypercoagulable states, especially the prothrombin gene 20210 mutation.[22] Genetic hypercoagulable states as etiologic factors are much more common in patients who are not cirrhotic but have portal vein, hepatic vein, and mesenteric vein thromboses.[23,24]

Despite the nearly universally elevated prothrombin time and thrombocytopenia in patients who have decompensated cirrhosis, DVT and PE do occur in this population. With the advent of better medical, procedural, and transplantation therapies in modern times, patients who have cirrhosis have significantly longer life spans than previously.[25,26] This increased survival is associated with more disability, a higher prevalence of obesity, longer survival with malignancy, and more procedural and surgical interventions, often in patients who have significant decompensation. All of these factors combine to give patients who have cirrhosis many similar risk factors for DVT/PE to general medicine patients. Retrospective series have estimated the incidence of DVT/PE in the hospitalized patients who have cirrhosis to be more than 0.5%[27] per hospitalization (see **Fig. 1** and **Fig. 2**). Unsurprisingly, laboratory coagulation parameters, including the international normalized ratio and platelet count, were not predictive of these events. Further study is needed to determine which patients are at highest risk for DVT/PE and which prophylactic interventions are appropriate.

Microvascular thrombotic disease

The consequences of macrovascular hypercoagulation may be the most easily diagnosed disorders, but mounting evidence shows that microvascular thrombosis may account for many other associated disease processes in patients who have cirrhosis. Portopulmonary hypertension may be one such process. Many patients who have cirrhosis have mildly elevated pulmonary artery pressures, but 3% to 8% have moderate

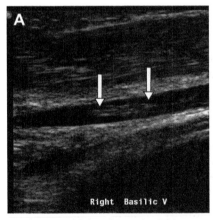 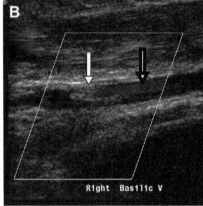

Fig.1. Ultrasound (*A*) and Doppler (*B*) images of a 33-year-old woman who had nonalcoholic steatohepatitis with cirrhosis and acute decompensation with a spontaneous right basilic vein thrombosis (*white arrows*). The thrombus was nonocclusive and some flow occurred in the vessel (*B; dark arrow*). At thrombosis, her international normalized ratio was 4.7, prothrombin time was 47 seconds, and platelet count was 91,000/μL.

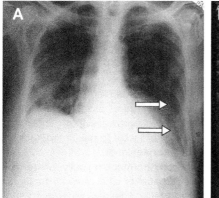
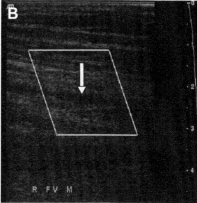

Fig. 2. Chest radiograph (A) and Doppler (B) ultrasound images of a 75-year-old man who had nonalcoholic steatohepatitis with cirrhosis and a recently diagnosed hepatocellular carcinoma who presented with a pulmonary embolism. Chest radiograph showed a left hydropneumothorax (A; *arrows*) and ultrasound showed a noncompressible right femoral vein without flow consistent with deep vein thrombosis (B; *arrows*). At presentation, his international normalized ratio was 1.9 and prothrombin time was 22 seconds.

to severely elevated mean pressures greater than 35 mm Hg. When no other cause can be found, these patients are at a significantly increased risk for death compared with other patients who have cirrhosis.[28]

Although definitive data are lacking, autopsy studies have suggested a microvascular thrombotic process as a cause.[29] Potential pathophysiologic mechanisms include a loss of endothelial barrier function followed by activation of coagulation with concurrent exposure of the smooth muscle layer to vasoconstrictive, proliferative, and thrombotic signals, and eventual development of a plexogenic arteriopathy.[30] Similar arguments have been raised in type 2 hepatorenal syndrome[31] and in the vascular permeability believed to be a possible mechanism for spontaneous bacterial peritonitis.[32]

Finally, significant evidence shows that chronic intrahepatic microthrombosis plays a key role in the initiation and progression of fibrosis and the eventual development of atrophy. This process has been termed *parenchymal extinction*[33] (see also article by Anstee and colleagues elsewhere in this issue). Aggregation of activated platelets is closely related to tissue damage in various inflammatory gastrointestinal disorders[34] and a similar process may occur in cirrhotic livers.[35] The process of parenchymal extinction has been most thoroughly studied in cardiac (congestive) hepatopathy[36] and nonalcoholic steatohepatitis,[37] but the general theory of progression of fibrosis through parenchymal extinction may explain many forms of cirrhosis-associated atrophy. Similar evidence supports a hypercoagulable state promoting more aggressive fibrosis in hepatitis C infection[38–41] and nonalcoholic steatohepatitis.[37,42,43] These data suggest that targeted interventions preventing the hypercoagulable state at the microvascular level may be able to prevent or delay progression of cirrhosis in many disease states.

SUMMARY

The coagulopathy of liver disease is extraordinarily complex and unpredictable, especially with conventional tests such as prothrombin time and international normalized ratio. Despite clear evidence of an increased bleeding tendency in patients who have cirrhosis, many circumstances also promote local and systemic hypercoagulable states, and it is clear that so-called "auto-anticoagulation" in cirrhosis is a myth. The consequences of hypercoagulability include the obvious morbidity and mortality of portal vein thrombosis, DVT, and PE, but possibly also other end-organ syndromes, such as portopulmonary hypertension, hepatorenal syndrome, and spontaneous bacterial peritonitis. The more subtle contribution could also be responsible for progression of early fibrosis to decompensated cirrhosis. Future clinical and laboratory research is needed to elucidate specific mechanistic pathways that might be lead to local hypercoagulation, including prothrombotic factor persistence, abnormal platelet activation, and inappropriate intravascular coagulation.

If the responsible mechanisms could be targeted pharmacologically, prevention of microvascular and macrovascular thrombosis in patients who have cirrhosis could lead to a significant impact on morbidity and mortality. Clinical research should focus on developing better testing modalities to determine which patients are susceptible to hypercoagulation, and thus avoid increasing the bleeding risk unnecessarily in patients not likely to benefit from antithrombotic therapies. Clinical research should also investigate prophylactic measures for macrovascular complications, such as portal vein thrombosis, DVT, and PE. With careful study design, it is now feasible to consider investigation of anticoagulation, especially antiplatelet agents, in preventing the progression of early-stage fibrosis in nonalcoholic steatohepatitis and hepatitis C.

REFERENCES

1. Lisman T, Leebeek FW, de Groot PG. Haemostatic abnormalities in patients with liver disease. J Hepatol 2002;37(2):280–7.
2. Vukovich T, Teufelsbauer H, Fritzer M, et al. Hemostasis activation in patients with liver cirrhosis. Thromb Res 1995;77(3):271–8.
3. Furchgott RF, Zawadzki JV. The obligatory role of endothelial cells in the relaxation of arterial smooth muscle by acetylcholine. Nature 1980;288(5789):373–6.
4. Moncada S, Higgs EA. Molecular mechanisms and therapeutic strategies related to nitric oxide. FASEB J 1995;9(13):1319–30.
5. Hamberg M, Svensson J, Samuelsson B. Thromboxanes: a new group of biologically active compounds derived from prostaglandin endoperoxides. Proc Natl Acad Sci U S A 1975;72(8):2994–8.
6. Marcus AJ, Broekman MJ, Pinsky DJ. COX inhibitors and thromboregulation. N Engl J Med 2002;347(13):1025–6.
7. Rubanyi GM, Polokoff MA. Endothelins: molecular biology, biochemistry, pharmacology, physiology, and pathophysiology. Pharmacol Rev 1994;46(3):325–415.
8. Marcus AJ, Broekman MJ, Drosopoulos JH, et al. Metabolic control of excessive extracellular nucleotide accumulation by CD39/ecto-nucleotidase-1: implications for ischemic vascular diseases. J Pharmacol Exp Ther 2003;305(1):9–16.
9. Artiko V, Obradovic V, Petrovic M, et al. Hepatic radionuclide angiography and Doppler ultrasonography in the detection and assessment of vascular disturbances in the portal system. Hepatogastroenterology 2007;54(75):892–7.
10. Ferguson JW, Dover AR, Chia S, et al. Inducible nitric oxide synthase activity contributes to the regulation of peripheral vascular tone in patients with cirrhosis and ascites. Gut 2006;55(4):542–6.
11. Moore K, Wendon J, Frazer M, et al. Plasma endothelin immunoreactivity in liver disease and the hepatorenal syndrome. N Engl J Med 1992;327(25):1774–8.

12. Ferro D, Quintarelli C, Lattuada A, et al. High plasma levels of von Willebrand factor as a marker of endothelial perturbation in cirrhosis: relationship to endotoxemia. Hepatology 1996;23(6):1377–83.

13. Kerr R, Newsome P, Germain L, et al. Effects of acute liver injury on blood coagulation. J Thromb Haemost 2003;1(4):754–9.

14. Tripodi A, Salerno F, Chantarangkul V, et al. Evidence of normal thrombin generation in cirrhosis despite abnormal conventional coagulation tests. Hepatology 2005;41(3):553–8.

15. Violi F, Ferro D, Basili S, et al. Prognostic value of clotting and fibrinolytic systems in a follow-up of 165 liver cirrhotic patients. CALC Group. Hepatology 1995;22(1):96–100.

16. Violi F, Ferro D, Basili S, et al. Hyperfibrinolysis resulting from clotting activation in patients with different degrees of cirrhosis. The CALC Group. Coagulation Abnormalities in Liver Cirrhosis. Hepatology 1993;17(1):78–83.

17. Violi F, Ferro D, Basili S, et al. Association between low-grade disseminated intravascular coagulation and endotoxemia in patients with liver cirrhosis. Gastroenterology 1995;109(2):531–9.

18. Hu KQ, Yu AS, Tiyyagura L, et al. Hyperfibrinolytic activity in hospitalized cirrhotic patients in a referral liver unit. Am J Gastroenterol 2001;96(5):1581–6.

19. Oka K, Tanaka K. Intravascular coagulation in autopsy cases with liver diseases. Thromb Haemost 1979;42(2):564–70.

20. Nonami T, Yokoyama I, Iwatsuki S, et al. The incidence of portal vein thrombosis at liver transplantation. Hepatology 1992;16(5):1195–8.

21. Okuda K, Ohnishi K, Kimura K, et al. Incidence of portal vein thrombosis in liver cirrhosis. An angiographic study in 708 patients. Gastroenterology 1985;89(2):279–86.

22. Amitrano L, Guardascione MA, Brancaccio V, et al. Risk factors and clinical presentation of portal vein thrombosis in patients with liver cirrhosis. J Hepatol 2004;40(5):736–41.

23. Murad SD, Valla DC, de Groen PC, et al. Pathogenesis and treatment of Budd-Chiari syndrome combined with portal vein thrombosis. Am J Gastroenterol 2006;101(1):83–90.

24. Kocher G, Himmelmann A. Portal vein thrombosis (PVT): a study of 20 non-cirrhotic cases. Swiss Med Wkly 2005;135(25-26):372–6.

25. Carbonell N, Pauwels A, Serfaty L, et al. Improved survival after variceal bleeding in patients with cirrhosis over the past two decades. Hepatology 2004;40(3):652–9.

26. Sorensen HT, Thulstrup AM, Mellemkjar L, et al. Long-term survival and cause-specific mortality in patients with cirrhosis of the liver: a nationwide cohort study in Denmark. J Clin Epidemiol 2003;56(1):88–93.

27. Northup PG, McMahon MM, Ruhl AP, et al. Coagulopathy does not fully protect hospitalized cirrhosis patients from peripheral venous thromboembolism. Am J Gastroenterol 2006;101(7):1524–8.

28. Kawut SM, Taichman DB, Ahya VN, et al. Hemodynamics and survival of patients with portopulmonary hypertension. Liver Transpl 2005;11(9):1107–11.

29. Mantz F, Craige E. Portal axis thrombosis with spontaneous portocaval shunt and cor pulmonale. Arch Pathol 1951;52:91–7.

30. Fallon MB. Mechanisms of pulmonary vascular complications of liver disease: hepatopulmonary syndrome. J Clin Gastroentero. 2005;39(4 Suppl 2):S138–42.

31. Mandal AK, Lansing M, Fahmy A. Acute tubular necrosis in hepatorenal syndrome: an electron microscopy study. Am J Kidney Dis 1982;2(3):363–74.

32. Nagler A, Hayek T, Brenner B, et al. Recurrent spontaneous bacterial peritonitis in a patient with polycythemia vera. Am J Hematol 1988;29(1):54–5.
33. Wanless IR, Wong F, Blendis LM, et al. Hepatic and portal vein thrombosis in cirrhosis: possible role in development of parenchymal extinction and portal hypertension. Hepatology 1995;21(5):1238–47.
34. Kayo S, Ikura Y, Suekane T, et al. Close association between activated platelets and neutrophils in the active phase of ulcerative colitis in humans. Inflamm Bowel Dis 2006;12(8):727–35.
35. Ikura Y, Morimoto H, Ogami M, et al. Expression of platelet-derived growth factor and its receptor in livers of patients with chronic liver disease. J Gastroenterol 1997;32(4):496–501.
36. Wanless IR, Liu JJ, Butany J. Role of thrombosis in the pathogenesis of congestive hepatic fibrosis (cardiac cirrhosis). Hepatology 1995;21(5):1232–7.
37. Wanless IR, Shiota K. The pathogenesis of nonalcoholic steatohepatitis and other fatty liver diseases: a four-step model including the role of lipid release and hepatic venular obstruction in the progression to cirrhosis. Semin Liver Dis 2004;24(1):99–106.
38. Wright M, Goldin R, Hellier S, et al. Factor V Leiden polymorphism and the rate of fibrosis development in chronic hepatitis C virus infection. Gut 2003;52(8):1206–10.
39. Poujol-Robert A, Boelle PY, Poupon R, et al. Factor V Leiden as a risk factor for cirrhosis in chronic hepatitis C. Hepatology 2004;39(4):1174–5.
40. Prieto J, Yuste JR, Beloqui O, et al. Anticardiolipin antibodies in chronic hepatitis C: implication of hepatitis C virus as the cause of the antiphospholipid syndrome. Hepatology 1996;23(2):199–204.
41. Goulding C, O'Brien C, Egan H, et al. The impact of inherited prothrombotic risk factors on individuals chronically infected with hepatitis C virus from a single source. Journal of Viral Hepatitis 2007;14(4):255–9.
42. Assy N, Bekirov I, Mejritsky Y, et al. Association between thrombotic risk factors and extent of fibrosis in patients with non-alcoholic fatty liver diseases. World J Gastroenterol 2005;11(37):5834–9.
43. Villanova N, Moscatiello S, Ramilli S, et al. Endothelial dysfunction and cardiovascular risk profile in nonalcoholic fatty liver disease. Hepatology 2005;42(2):473–80.

Parenchymal Extinction: Coagulation and Hepatic Fibrogenesis

Quentin M. Anstee, BSc, MBBS, PhD, MRCP[a],[*],
Mark Wright, BSc, MBBS, PhD, MRCP[b],
Robert Goldin, MD, FRCPath[c],
Mark R. Thursz, MBBS, MD, FRCP[a]

KEYWORDS

- Liver • Fibrosis • Thrombophilia
- Factor V Leiden • Coagulation

The development of hepatic fibrosis following chronic liver injury, irrespective of etiology, may be influenced by the interaction of host genetic factors, the pathogen, and other coincidental environmental influences. Hepatic fibrogenesis is essentially wound healing on a whole organ scale.[1] The process is triggered by tissue damage and continues until the lesion is healed. If the damage persists or is fluctuant, the repair process persists. Removal of the underlying etiology before the development of cirrhosis and liver failure is the primary therapeutic goal in treating liver disease. If this cannot be achieved, a secondary goal is to inhibit liver fibrosis; however, there are no effective well-tolerated drugs available. The mechanism by which fibrosis and the progression to cirrhosis occur is an area of intense research interest.

The progression of fibrosis in patients with chronic hepatitis C virus (HCV) infection seems to be steady and persistent and has been studied more intensely than many other etiologies. It is a good model in which to investigate factors that influence rate of progression. Cross-sectional studies in European patients with HCV infection have determined a number of host factors that influence the rate of disease progression to cirrhosis.[2,3] The median time from infection to cirrhosis in these studies was 30 to 35 years (**Fig. 1**).[2,3] Subsequently, disease progresses to hepatic decompensation (4%–9.5% per annum) or hepatocellular carcinoma (1.4%–5% per annum). Annual transition from cirrhosis to death or transplant is 2% to 6%.[4–7]

[a] Department of Academic Medicine, St Mary's Hospital Campus, Imperial College London, 10th Floor, QEQM Building, Praed Street, London W2 1PG, UK
[b] Department of Hepatology, Southampton General Hospital, Southampton, UK
[c] Department of Histopathology, St Mary's Hospital Campus, Imperial College London, 10th Floor, QEQM Building, Praed Street, London W2 1PG, UK
* Corresponding author.
E-mail address: q.anstee@imperial.ac.uk (Q.M. Anstee).

Clin Liver Dis 13 (2009) 117–126
doi:10.1016/j.cld.2008.09.013
1089-3261/08/$ – see front matter © 2009 Elsevier Inc. All rights reserved.

liver.theclinics.com

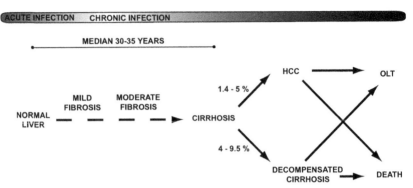

Fig. 1. Natural history of chronic hepatitis C infection. HCC, hepatocellular carcinoma; OLT, orthotopic liver transplant.

Male gender, age at infection, and alcohol consumption are determinants of accelerated fibrosis progression in HCV infection.[2,8] Such factors only account for a fraction (17%–29%) of the interpatient variability that is observed in clinical practice.[2,9] Cohort studies have identified additional genetic and environmental cofactors that influence the rate of hepatic fibrogenesis (eg, body mass index and the presence of hepatic steatosis). Available evidence suggests that coagulation status should be added to this list.

A ROLE FOR CLOTTING IN HEPATIC FIBROGENESIS
Microthrombi and Hepatic Damage in Animal Models

The first evidence of a role for coagulation in the pathogenesis of liver disease came from studies examining the effects of acute murine hepatitis virus infection in C3HeB/FeJ and Balb/cJ mice. Corrosion casts of the hepatic microvasculature demonstrated microthombi associated with areas of tissue necrosis.[10–12] Disease severity in this hepatic infection model is strongly related to the presence of microthrombi, an effect that may be mediated by Fgl2/Fibroleukin (a prothrombinase whose expression on the surface of hepatic endothelial cells is induced by viral infections including hepatitis B).[13]

Acute and chronic carbon tetrachloride–induced liver injury also stimulate hepatic deposition of fibrin and fibrinogen within the microcirculation.[14] More recently, studies in the same model indicate that accelerated hepatic fibrogenesis occurs in animals carrying the prothrombotic factor V Leiden (FvL) mutation.[15] A parallel literature reports similar results in the bleomycin inhalation mouse model of pulmonary fibrosis.[16]

Epidemiologic and Clinical Evidence

Wanless and colleagues[17,18] first reported the presence of thrombi within the hepatic microvasculature of patients with cirrhosis. Using a cohort of Greek patients with hepatitis B and hepatitis C, Papatheodoridis and colleagues[19] demonstrated that patients with advanced fibrosis (Ishak stage 4–6) were significantly more likely to have thrombophilia related to a deficiency of protein C, antithrombin III, and plasminogen. In addition, the HENCORE collaboration published data demonstrating that heterozygote carriage of the FvL mutation was associated with an odds ratio of 3.28 for rapid progression to cirrhosis in a European white HCV population.[9] Subsequently, this was validated in an independent patient population.[20] Furthermore, protein C deficiency, increased expression of factor VIII, and hyperhomocysteinemia have also been linked to advanced HCV fibrosis.[21] One study, examining the effect of FvL carriage in a cohort of women infected by HCV-contaminated anti-D immunoglobulin, did not find an association between fibrosis and prothrombotic status.[22] Overall fibrosis stage in this cohort was extremely low, however, and whereas the effect of FvL carriage in the original article was most pronounced in males,[9] the cohort studied was all female.[22]

Although studies in humans indicate that a hypercoagulant, prothrombotic state promotes accelerated fibrogenesis, further support to the role of coagulation in hepatic fibrogenesis comes from studies examining the natural history of HCV-infected hemophiliac patients without HIV coinfection. These suggest a slow progression of liver fibrosis with only 3% (95% confidence interval, 0.4%–6%) having liver-related deaths in one study. This comprised 6 of 185 HIV-negative patients, 5 of whom were know also to take excess alcohol; one died following liver biopsy.[23]

PATHOGENIC MECHANISMS

Based on current literature, two complimentary hypotheses may be proposed that explain how activity of the coagulation cascade may affect changes in the rate of hepatic fibrosis progression. Both are biologically plausible and support a role for the coagulation system in the control of tissue repair and remodeling.

Parenchymal Extinction: Intrahepatic Microthrombi Causing Tissue Ischemia and Fibrosis

Large thrombi occluding the hepatic vein are generally accepted as a cause of hepatic fibrosis in Budd-Chiari syndrome.[24] Wanless and colleagues[17,18] observed that the extent and distribution of microthrombi within branches of the hepatic vein and portal vein correlated with progression of hepatic fibrosis in a number of pathologies including HCV, hepatitis B virus, primary biliary cirrhosis, alcoholic liver disease, and cardiac cirrhosis. Microthrombi may also contribute to liver allograft rejection[25] and the development of thrombocytopenia in cirrhosis.[26] Based on these observations Wanless and colleagues[17,18] proposed that microinfarcts were the critical event in the genesis of fibrous septa and hence cirrhosis. He postulated that occlusive thrombi, initiated by intimal injury caused by adjacent hepatic necroinflammation, form within branches of the hepatic vein and portal vein and disrupt the flow of blood (**Fig. 2**). Obliteration of small hepatic and portal venules causes congestion and reactive hyperemia. Together with vascular endothelial growth factor–induced angiogenesis, this leads to an imbalance between sinusoidal inflow and outflow leading to congestion, exudation, and hemorrhage.[17,18] The consequent sinusoidal injury and tissue ischemia causes hepatocyte apoptosis and collapse of the region between the central veins and their adjacent portal tracts.[17,18] The resulting parenchymal extinction lesion may be defined as the irreversible loss of contiguous hepatocytes from a region, and replacement by fibrous tissue. Cirrhosis occurs when small areas of parenchymal extinction accumulate and become confluent.[27]

The same group has subsequently reported evidence of parenchymal extinction in patients with non-alcoholic fatty liver disease (NAFLD) and a rabbit model of fibrosing steatohepatitis induced by a combination of diethylstilbestrol injections (a synthetic estrogen that is associated with an increased risk of thrombosis) and a high-cholesterol diet.[28,29]

Direct Stellate Cell Activation: Thrombin-Mediated Hepatic Stellate Cell Activation by Protease Activated Receptors-1

The alternative hypothesis centers on thrombin's wide range of biologic activity beyond the coagulation cascade and so does not necessarily require the development of intrahepatic thrombosis to explain the increase in tissue fibrosis. Thrombin is

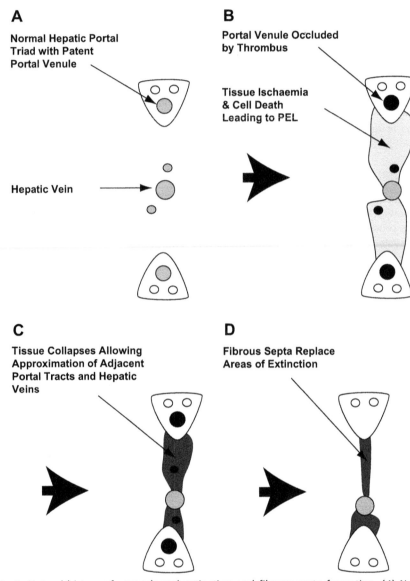

Fig. 2. Natural history of parenchymal extinction and fibrous septa formation. (*A*) Normal liver with patent portal and hepatic veins. (*B*) Inflammatory injury causes venous thrombosis (*black circles*). The consequent hepatocyte ischemia and death leads to parenchymal extinction. (*C*) Extinction allows tissue to collapse so that adjacent portal tracts and hepatic veins are approximated. (*D*) Regions of parenchymal extinction are replaced by fibrous septa. The obliterated venules are no longer evident. PEL, parenchymal extinction lesion.

a serine protease and is able to signal to a variety of cell types by a family of G-protein coupled protease-activated receptors (PAR). Cleavage of the amino-terminal extracellular domain of the PAR receptor unmasks a new *N*-terminus tethered ligand that effects transmembrane signaling. Four PAR receptors have been described. PAR-1 and PAR-3 are considered to have high affinity for thrombin activation, whereas

PAR-4 has a reduced affinity and PAR-2 is resistant to thrombin activation.[30] Fibro-blasts and stellate cells from both humans and rodents have been shown to express PAR-1; rodents also expressed PAR-4, although this was not tested in human studies.[31,32] Acting by PAR-1, thrombin is chemotactic for monocytes and mitogenic for smooth muscle cells, fibroblasts, and hepatic stellate cells.

In vitro studies using selective PAR-1 and PAR-4 agonists demonstrate that these are able to induce stellate cell activation.[31] Activation of PAR-1 by thrombin-mediated proteolytic cleavage leads to rapid stellate cell activation and secretion of extracellular matrix proteins, tissue remodeling, and fibrogenesis (**Fig. 3**).[31–33] Several studies have established that hepatic PAR-1 expression is increased during acute and chronic hep-atitis[32] and in liver injury caused by bile duct ligation,[31] sensitizing stellate cells to thrombin-mediated activation. These observations suggest that substrate (PAR-1)

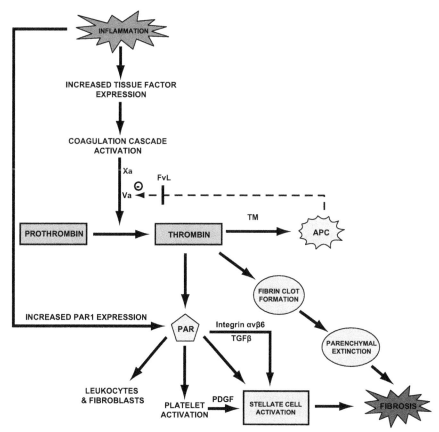

Fig. 3. PAR-1–mediated actions of thrombin in stellate cell activation. Inflammation within the hepatic parenchyma increases expression of tissue factor, a key initiator of the coagula-tion cascade, and the thrombin receptor, PAR-1. Inflammation primes both the generation of thrombin and its down-stream signaling activity. In the presence of the FvL mutation, the normal thrombin-thrombomodulin negative feedback loop by activated protein C, which limits thrombin production, is ineffective. This allows thrombin generation to proceed unchecked in a hepatic environment that is already sensitized for PAR-1–mediated stellate cell activation both directly and by platelet-released platelet-derived growth factor. APC, activated protein C; PDGF, platelet-derived growth factor; TGF, transforming growth factor; TM, thrombomodulin.

availability ceases to be a rate limiting factor at sites of inflammation. A prothrombotic state, characterized by an increase in the basal levels of thrombin generation within the circulation, may contribute to fibrogenesis by enhancing direct activation of stellate cells. In this way increased thrombin production, caused by failure of the thrombin-thrombomodulin negative feedback loop by activated protein C, as occurs in carriage of the FvL mutation, could amplify PAR-1 signaling (see **Fig. 3**). This model for the role of thrombin and FvL in the genesis of hepatic fibrosis is supported by studies that demonstrate fibrosis is ameliorated by administration of a PAR-1 antagonist.[31] Similarly, PAR-1 knockout mice are protected from bleomycin inhalation–induced pulmonary fibrosis.[34]

Platelets in mice express PAR-3 and PAR-4, whereas in humans PAR-1 and PAR-4 expression has been demonstrated.[35] In addition to direct PAR-mediated stellate cell activation, thrombin can also stimulate platelet degranulation and the release of platelet-derived growth factor (PDGF), another potent stellate cell activator, by the PAR receptor (see **Fig. 3**).[36] Further, activation of PAR-1 has been shown to facilitate the $\alpha_v\beta_6$ integrin-dependent posttranslational activation of latent transforming growth factor-β, a key mediator of fibrogenesis.[37] Recently published data using two separate cohorts of HCV patients also demonstrate a more rapid rate of hepatic fibrosis is associated with carriage of a Δ-1426C/T transition mutation in the 5' regulatory region of the PAR-1 gene, further supporting the role of thrombin-mediated signaling in hepatic fibrogenesis.[38] Taken together, these place thrombin-mediated PAR signaling as an effector of direct stellate cell activation, indirect stellate cell activation by platelet-derived growth factor release, and posttranslational transforming growth factor-β activation.

Clearly, the parenchymal extinction hypothesis and the PAR-1–mediated stellate cell activation hypothesis are not mutually exclusive. Indeed, venulitis resulting from adjacent parenchymal inflammation may result in thrombosis more readily in the presence of a thrombophilic condition. Although data supporting the role of the coagulation cascade in driving fibrosis are strong, experimental data supporting parenchymal extinction remain sparse.

POTENTIAL THERAPEUTIC IMPLICATIONS

A corollary of the association between hypercoagulation and increased fibrosis is that interference with either the generation of thrombin or its downstream activity may reduce hepatic fibrosis. Several studies support this hypothesis.

Therapeutic Studies in Animal Models

Administration of a PAR-1 antagonist reduces hepatic fibrosis and stellate cell activation in the rat bile duct ligation model.[31] It has been demonstrated that carbon tetrachloride–induced hepatic fibrosis in C57BL/6 mice may be slowed by concomitant administration of coumarin (warfarin).[15] The synthetic thrombin inhibitor SSR182289 has also demonstrated decreased fibrogenesis compared with controls in carbon tetrachloride–exposed rats.[39] Similar results have also been reported in this and other models of liver damage using low-molecular-weight heparin.[40,41] Studies in the rabbit model of fibrosing steatohepatitis induced by a combination of diethylstilbestrol injections and a high-cholesterol diet have reported that concomitant administration of dipyridamole (a pyrimidopyridine derivative with antiplatelet and vasodilator properties) reduced hepatic fibrosis.[28] Aerosolized heparin or urokinase are similarly effective in ameliorating bleomycin-induced pulmonary fibrosis.[42]

Therapeutic Effects in Humans

Although existing data do not support the routine use of therapeutic anticoagulation as an antifibrotic therapy, it is becoming evident that activity of the coagulation cascade has a profound influence on tissue fibrogenesis. This has potentially significant clinical implications and offers the prospect of novel therapeutic approaches. To date, one small study suggesting efficacy of low-molecular-weight heparin as an antifibrotic in patients with chronic hepatitis B virus has been reported;[43] however, further trials are needed. Pursuing an analogous hypothesis, a Japanese group has also reported reduced mortality from a pilot study of coumarin (warfarin) treatment in patients with idiopathic pulmonary fibrosis.[44]

The choice of agent and clinical efficacy need to be evaluated fully in clinical trials. These require careful selection of agent and study population. Suitable agents may include antiplatelet drugs, such as dipyridamole, coumarins, and direct thrombin inhibitors. The latter are small molecules, which bind directly to the catalytic site of both clot bound and free thrombin and give more consistent anticoagulant responses without the need for monitoring. Despite the withdrawal by the Food and Drug Administration of ximelagatran because of raised transaminases, there are several others (eg, dabigatran etexilate) at the phase 3 trial stage for prevention of venous thromboembolism that may be suitable.[45]

Given the risk of hemorrhage once portal hypertension is established, antithrombotic therapy may be best used in the precirrhotic patient. Because most human studies on fibrogenesis rate have been conducted in patients with chronic HCV infection, this represents a suitable group for therapeutic trials. Because of intolerance of the current interferon-based treatments or failure of response there is an expanding cohort of patients with a progressive fibrotic liver disease requiring alternative therapeutic strategies. Trials in this group of patients may be challenging because of the slowly progressive nature of HCV and the need for frequent biopsies. Patients infected with HCV who are post–liver transplant represent a more appropriate group because their liver disease tends to progress rapidly and frequent biopsies are taken as part of follow-up protocol. A United Kingdom–based multicenter trial (WAFT-C) examining the efficacy of coumarin as an antifibrotic in the posttransplant chronic HCV population is currently underway.

SUMMARY

The development of hepatic fibrosis following chronic liver injury may be influenced by the interaction between host genetic factors, the pathogen, and other coincidental environmental influences. Observations that hepatic inflammation and established cirrhosis were associated with the presence of thrombi within the hepatic microvasculature and fibrin-fibrinogen deposition led to epidemiologic studies examining prothrombotic risk factors and rate of hepatic fibrosis. Carriage of the FvL mutation, protein C deficiency, and increased expression of factor VIII were associated with rapid progression to cirrhosis in chronic HCV. Based on current literature, two complimentary hypotheses may be proposed that explain how activity of the coagulation cascade may influence the rate of hepatic fibrogenesis: tissue ischemia and parenchymal extinction; and direct thrombin-mediated stellate cell activation by PAR-1 cleavage. Current clinical data and in vivo models support a role for coagulation cascade activity in hepatic fibrosis mediated by downstream events of thrombin activation. The corollary of an association between hypercoagulation and increased fibrosis is that interference with either the generation of thrombin or its downstream activity may reduce hepatic fibrosis, and there are substantial implications for future therapeutic intervention. Clinical studies are already underway to address this possibility.

REFERENCES

1. Iredale JP. Models of liver fibrosis: exploring the dynamic nature of inflammation and repair in a solid organ. J Clin Invest 2007;117(3):539–48.
2. Poynard T, Bedossa P, Opolon P. Natural history of liver fibrosis progression in patients with chronic hepatitis C. The OBSVIRC, METAVIR, CLINIVIR, and DOS-VIRC groups. Lancet 1997;349(9055):825–32.
3. Wright M, Goldin R, Fabre A, et al. Measurement and determinants of the natural history of liver fibrosis in hepatitis C virus infection: a cross sectional and longitudinal study. Gut 2003;52(4):574–9.
4. Fattovich G, Giustina G, Degos F, et al. Morbidity and mortality in compensated cirrhosis type C: a retrospective follow-up study of 384 patients. Gastroenterology 1997;112(2):463–72.
5. Serfaty L, Aumaitre H, Chazouilleres O, et al. Determinants of outcome of compensated hepatitis C virus-related cirrhosis. Hepatology 1998;27(5):1435–40.
6. Hu KQ, Tong MJ. The long-term outcomes of patients with compensated hepatitis C virus-related cirrhosis and history of parenteral exposure in the United States. Hepatology 1999;29(4):1311–6.
7. Niederau C, Lange S, Heintges T, et al. Prognosis of chronic hepatitis C: results of a large, prospective cohort study. Hepatology 1998;28(6):1687–95.
8. Poynard T, Ratziu V, Charlotte F, et al. Rates and risk factors of liver fibrosis progression in patients with chronic hepatitis c. J Hepatol 2001;34(5):730–9.
9. Wright M, Goldin R, Hellier S, et al. Factor V Leiden polymorphism and the rate of fibrosis development in chronic hepatitis C virus infection. Gut 2003;52(8):1206–10.
10. MacPhee PJ, Dindzans VJ, Fung LS, et al. Acute and chronic changes in the microcirculation of the liver in inbred strains of mice following infection with mouse hepatitis virus type 3. Hepatology 1985;5(4):649–60.
11. MacPhee PJ, Schmidt EE, Keown PA, et al. Microcirculatory changes in livers of mice infected with murine hepatitis virus: evidence from microcorrosion casts and measurements of red cell velocity. Microvasc Res 1988;36(2):140–9.
12. Levy GA, MacPhee PJ, Fung LS, et al. The effect of mouse hepatitis virus infection on the microcirculation of the liver. Hepatology 1983;3(6):964–73.
13. Marsden PA, Ning Q, Fung LS, et al. The Fgl2/fibroleukin prothrombinase contributes to immunologically mediated thrombosis in experimental and human viral hepatitis. J Clin Invest 2003;112(1):58–66.
14. Neubauer K, Knittel T, Armbrust T, et al. Accumulation and cellular localization of fibrinogen/fibrin during short-term and long-term rat liver injury. Gastroenterology 1995;108(4):1124–35.
15. Anstee QM, Wright M, Goldin R, et al. Coagulation status modulates hepatic fibrosis: implications for the development of novel therapies. Journal of Thrombosis & Haemostasis 2008;6(8):1336–43.
16. Xu Z, Westrick RJ, Shen YC, et al. Pulmonary fibrosis is increased in mice carrying the factor V Leiden mutation following bleomycin injury. Thromb Haemost 2001;85(3):441–4.
17. Wanless IR, Wong F, Blendis LM, et al. Hepatic and portal vein thrombosis in cirrhosis: possible role in development of parenchymal extinction and portal hypertension. Hepatology 1995;21(5):1238–47.
18. Wanless IR, Liu JJ, Butany J. Role of thrombosis in the pathogenesis of congestive hepatic fibrosis (cardiac cirrhosis). Hepatology 1995;21(5):1232–7.
19. Papatheodoridis GV, Papakonstantinou E, Andrioti E, et al. Thrombotic risk factors and extent of liver fibrosis in chronic viral hepatitis. Gut 2003;52(3):404–9.

20. Poujol-Robert A, Boelle PY, Poupon R, et al. Factor V Leiden as a risk factor for cirrhosis in chronic hepatitis C. Hepatology 2004;39(4):1174–5.
21. Poujol-Robert A, Rosmorduc O, Serfaty L, et al. Genetic and acquired thrombotic factors in chronic hepatitis C. Am J Gastroenterol 2004;99(3):527–31.
22. Goulding C, O'Brien C, Egan H, et al. The impact of inherited prothrombotic risk factors on individuals chronically infected with hepatitis C virus from a single source. J Viral Hepat 2007;14(4):255–9.
23. Yee TT, Griffioen A, Sabin CA, et al. The natural history of HCV in a cohort of haemophilic patients infected between 1961 and 1985. Gut 2000;47(6):845–51.
24. Tanaka M, Wanless IR. Pathology of the liver in Budd-Chiari syndrome: portal vein thrombosis and the histogenesis of veno-centric cirrhosis, veno-portal cirrhosis, and large regenerative nodules. Hepatology 1998;27(2):488–96.
25. Nakazawa Y, Jonsson JR, Walker NI, et al. Fibrous obliterative lesions of veins contribute to progressive fibrosis in chronic liver allograft rejection. Hepatology 2000;32(6):1240–7.
26. Ikura Y, Kitabayashi C, Nakagawa M, et al. Secondary parenchymal damages in cirrhotic livers associated with activated platelet aggregation in sinusoids. Hepatology 2007;46(4):579A.
27. Wanless IR. Pathogenesis of cirrhosis. J Gastroenterol Hepatol 2004;19(Suppl): S369–71.
28. Wanless IR, Belgiorno J, Huet PM. Hepatic sinusoidal fibrosis induced by cholesterol and stilbestrol in the rabbit: 1. Morphology and inhibition of fibrogenesis by dipyridamole. Hepatology 1996;24(4):855–64.
29. Wanless IR, Shiota K. The pathogenesis of nonalcoholic steatohepatitis and other fatty liver diseases: a four-step model including the role of lipid release and hepatic venular obstruction in the progression to cirrhosis. Semin Liver Dis 2004; 24(1):99–106.
30. Di CE. Thrombin interactions. Chest 2003;124(3 Suppl):11S–7S.
31. Fiorucci S, Antonelli E, Distrutti E, et al. PAR1 antagonism protects against experimental liver fibrosis: role of proteinase receptors in stellate cell activation. Hepatology 2004;39(2):365–75.
32. Marra F, DeFranco R, Grappone C, et al. Expression of the thrombin receptor in human liver: up-regulation during acute and chronic injury. Hepatology 1998; 27(2):462–71.
33. Gaca MD, Zhou X, Benyon RC. Regulation of hepatic stellate cell proliferation and collagen synthesis by proteinase-activated receptors. J Hepatol 2002;36(3): 362–9.
34. Howell DC, Johns RH, Lasky JA, et al. Absence of proteinase-activated receptor-1 signaling affords protection from bleomycin-induced lung inflammation and fibrosis. Am J Pathol 2005;166(5):1353–65.
35. Coughlin SR. Thrombin signalling and protease-activated receptors. Nature 2000;407(6801):258–64.
36. Friedman SL. Liver fibrosis: from bench to bedside. J Hepatol 2003;38(Suppl 1):S38–53.
37. Jenkins RG, Su X, Su G, et al. Ligation of protease-activated receptor 1 enhances alphavbeta6 integrin-dependent TGF-beta activation and promotes acute lung injury. J Clin Invest 2006;116(6):1606–14.
38. Martinelli A, Knapp S, Anstee Q, et al. Effect of a thrombin receptor (protease-activated receptor 1, PAR-1) gene polymorphism in chronic hepatitis C liver fibrosis. J Gastroenterol Hepatol 2008;23(9):1403–9.
39. Duplantier JG, Dubuisson L, Senant N, et al. A role for thrombin in liver fibrosis. Gut 2004;53(11):1682–7.

40. Abdel-Salam OM, Baiuomy AR, Ameen A, et al. A study of unfractionated and low molecular weight heparins in a model of cholestatic liver injury in the rat. Pharm Res 2005;51(1):59–67.
41. Abe W, Ikejima K, Lang T, et al. Low molecular weight heparin prevents hepatic fibrogenesis caused by carbon tetrachloride in the rat. J Hepatol 2007;46(2): 286–94.
42. Gunther A, Lubke N, Ermert M, et al. Prevention of bleomycin-induced lung fibrosis by aerosolization of heparin or urokinase in rabbits. Am J Respir Crit Care Med 2003;168(11):1358–65.
43. Shi J, Hao JH, Ren WH, et al. Effects of heparin on liver fibrosis in patients with chronic hepatitis B. World J Gastroenterol 2003;9(7):1611–4.
44. Kubo H, Nakayama K, Yanai M, et al. Anticoagulant therapy for idiopathic pulmonary fibrosis. Chest 2005;128(3):1475–82.
45. Eriksson BI, Dahl OE, Rosencher N, et al. Dabigatran etexilate versus enoxaparin for prevention of venous thromboembolism after total hip replacement: a randomised, double-blind, non-inferiority trial. Lancet 2007;370(9591):949–56.

Portal Vein Thrombosis and Budd–Chiari Syndrome

Paulo Lisboa Bittencourt, MD, PhD[a],*, Cláudia Alves Couto, MD, PhD[b], Daniel Dias Ribeiro, MD, PhD[b,c]

KEYWORDS

- Portal vein thrombosis • Budd–Chiari syndrome • Cirrhosis
- Thrombophilia • Portal hypertension

Portal vein thrombosis (PVT) and Budd–Chiari syndrome (BCS) are caused by thrombosis and/or obstruction of the extrahepatic portal veins and the hepatic venous outflow tract, respectively.[1–3] Several heterogeneous prothrombotic disorders may cause thrombosis of the portal and hepatic veins.[2,3] Venous thrombosis usually results from the convergence of vessel wall injury and/or venous stasis, known as local triggering factors, and the occurrence of acquired and/or inherited thrombophilia, also known as systemic prothrombotic risk factors.[4–6]

RISK FACTORS FOR PORTAL VEIN THROMBOSIS AND BUDD–CHIARI SYNDROME

Local risk factors are responsible for 30% to 40% of the cases of PVT, but they are rarely reported in subjects with primary BCS.[6,7] Inflammatory intra-abdominal disorders such as appendicitis and pancreatitis, postoperative complications of abdominal surgery, particularly splenectomy and surgical portosystemic shunts, and portal hypertension are recognized intra-abdominal risk factors for PVT (**Table 1**). In contrast, distinct *systemic prothrombotic risk* factors have been recognized in 60% to 70% of PVT and up to 90% of BCS (**Table 2**). All of these have been associated with an increased systemic predisposition to deep vein thrombosis and/or pulmonary embolism and more than one prothrombotic risk factor has been implicated in the pathogenesis of PVT and BCS in up to one third of the patients.[4,5,8–18]

Some risk factors are more frequently associated with one or another of those vascular disorders of the liver. In this respect, most of the cases of PVT are attributable to

[a] Unit of Gastroenterology and Hepatology, Portuguese Hospital, Salvador, Bahia, Brazil
[b] Alfa Gastroenterology Institute, Federal University of Minas Gerais, Belo Horizonte, Minas Gerais, Brazil
[c] Department of Hematology, Federal University of Minas Gerais, Belo Horizonte, Minas Gerais, Brazil
* Corresponding author. Rua Prof. Clementino Fraga 220/1901, Salvador, Bahia, Brazil, CEP 40170050.
E-mail address: plbbr@uol.com.br (P.L. Bittencourt).

Clin Liver Dis 13 (2009) 127–144
doi:10.1016/j.cld.2008.10.002
1089-3261/08/$ – see front matter © 2009 Elsevier Inc. All rights reserved.

Table 1
Local risk factors associated with portal vein thrombosis and Budd–Chiari syndrome

Portal Vein Thrombosis	Budd–Chiari Syndrome
Focal inflammatory lesions: neonatal omphalitis, diverticulitis, appendicitis, pancreatitis, duodenal ulcer, cholecystitis, tuberculous lymphadenitis, Crohn's disease, ulcerative colitis, cytomegalovirus hepatitis Injury to the portal venous system: splenectomy, colectomy, gastrectomy, cholecystectomy, liver transplantation, abdominal trauma, surgical portosystemic shunting, transjugular intrahepatic portosystemic shunt placement, cirrhosis	Invasion or encasement of inferior vena cava or hepatic veins by neoplasia, liver cysts, or abscess. Budd–Chiari syndrome in this setting can be designated as "secondary" to a local extrinsic factor such as neoplasm, cyst, or abscess, which causes external compression.

Adapted from Valla DC. The diagnosis and management of the Budd–Chiari syndrome: consensus and controversies. Hepatology 2003;38:793–803; and Janssen HL, Garcia-Pagan JC, Elias E, et al. Budd–Chiari syndrome: a review by an expert panel. J Hepatol 2003;38:364–71.

Philadelphia (Ph) chromosome negative myeloproliferative diseases (MPD), antiphospholipid syndrome, or distinct inherited prothrombotic disorders, such as protein S deficiency and prothrombin gene mutation (see **Table 2**).[7–10] There is a great geographic variation, but MPD is one of the most frequent disorders associated with

Table 2
Frequency of acquired and inherited systemic prothrombotic risk factors in patients with PVT, BCS, DVT, and healthy controls

Prothrombotic Disorders	PVT, %[a]	BCS, %[b]	DVT, %[c]	Healthy Subjects, %[c]
Myeloproliferative diseases[d]	14–35	28–47	NA	NA
Antiphospholipid syndrome	5–23	5–21	4–21	5
Factor V Leiden mutation	3–14	14–31	15–20	5–12
Factor II gene mutation	3–22	4–6	4–8	1
Protein C deficiency	0–9	0–13	3–6	0.2–0.5
Protein S deficiency	2–30	0–6	2	0.03–0.13
Antithrombin deficiency	0–4.5	0–4	0.5–7.5	0.02
C677T MTHFR gene mutations[e]	0–11	13–52	Variable	12–46
Hyperhomocysteinemia	NA	0–37	10–25	5–10
Elevated factor VIII	NA	NA	15–25	NA
Pregnancy	0–4	0–15	[f]	NA
Oral contraceptive use	0–48	7–55	[f]	NA
None	16–22	6–23	50	NA

Several patients had one or more overlapping prothrombotic risk factors.
Abbreviations: BCS, Budd–Chiari syndrome; DVT, deep vein thrombosis; MTHFR, methylene tetrahydrofolate reductase; NA, not applicable; PVT, portal vein thrombosis.
  [a] *Adapted from* Refs.[8–11,53,57]
  [b] *Adapted from* Refs.[9,10,12–15,36]
  [c] *Adapted from* Refs.[4,5,17]
  [d] Occult MPD was not investigated in most of the cohorts.
  [e] The presence of C677T MTHFR gene mutations without an increase in homocystein level is not a risk factor for DVT.
  [f] Accounts for a threefold increase in the relative risk for DVT.

PVT. In general, the prevalence of inherited thrombophilia is far less common in the East when compared with the West.[11,19,20]

Local risk factors account for only a small number of the cases of BCS, which can then be designated as "secondary" BCS (see **Table 1**). Most patients with BCS have a "primary" disorder and share one or more prothrombotic risk factors, mainly MPD, oral contraceptive use, factor V Leiden mutation, and antiphospholipid syndrome. Myeloproliferative disorders, particularly polycythemia vera, are observed in approximately half of the cases of BCS, but fewer than 10% of the subjects with overt MPD develop BCS.[13] There is also some geographic variation in the prevalence of acquired thrombophilia in patients with BCS. The use of oral contraceptives is related to BCS more frequently in Western, when compared with Eastern patients. On the other hand, poor sanitation has been associated with BCS, particularly with inferior vena cava (IVC) involvement in the Asian countries and poor socioeconomic status.[21]

EVALUATION OF THROMBOPHILIA, PORTAL VEIN THROMBOSIS, AND BUDD–CHIARI SYNDROME

Because of the high frequency of inherited and/or acquired prothrombotic disorders in patients with PVT and BCS, a systematic investigation of these risk factors is warranted and a formal hematological consultation is usually recomended, because the usual diagnostic criteria for those disorders cannot always be applied to subjects with underlying liver disease.[4,18,22,23]

Myeloproliferative diseases are the single most common group of disorders associated with PVT and BCS. In most cases, the Ph chromosome negative MPD can be classified as polycythemia vera, essential thrombocythemia or myelofibrosis. These diagnoses in patients with PVT and BCS, using the current World Health Organization criteria, may be misleading because of the presence of increased plasma volume and hypersplenism in the subjects with chronic liver disease (CLD) and portal hypertension. In this regard, detection of spontaneous endogenous erythrocyte colonies (EEC), determination of the somatic JAK2 V617F mutation,[13,24–27] and bone marrow biopsy to assess the presence of dystrophic megakariocytes has been used to diagnose MPD without typical phenotypic markers in subjects with and without CLD.[8,26] Based on the results of these assays, up to two thirds of the patients with either PVT or BCS were shown to have either overt or occult MPD.[28] However, some drawbacks associated with use of these parameters to diagnose occult MPD have to be highlighted.

The EEC assay is a nonstandardized labor-intensive method that is highly dependant on local laboratory expertise. It can yield negative results in subjects with clear-cut criteria for MPD and positive results in healthy subjects and patients with nonclonal polycythemia,[29] which limits its diagnostic accuracy for MPD.[29–32]

Recently, several investigators have identified an acquired mutation in the autoregulatory pseudokinase domain (JH2) of Janus kinase-2 (JAK2) gene in patients with MPD. One substitution of valine to phenylalanine at position 617 (V617F) was observed in 90% to 95% of the patients with polycythemia vera, 50% to 70% of the patients with essential thrombocythemia, and 40% to 50% of the patients with myelofibrosis.[33] Preliminary data have also suggested that MPD patients with JAK2 have an increased risk of thrombosis, hemorrhage, fibrosis, and cytoreductive treatment requirement when compared with their JAK2 negative counterparts;[34] however, data on the functional consequences of this mutation are still scarce. Noninvasive assessment of V617F JAK2 mutation for evaluation of MPD in patients with hepatic or splanchnic vein thrombosis is promising, but it should be emphasized that its presence is not sufficient for defining the MPD phenotype[23] and that V617F JAK2 mutation may be absent in a significant proportion of patients with PVT and BCS with overt MPD.[35,36]

Antiphospholipid antibodies syndrome (APS) is seen in 5% to 23% of the patients with PVT or BCS. The antiphospholipid antibodies are a group of autoantibodies that target phospholipid binding proteins, including lupus anticoagulant, IgM and IgG anticardiolipin, and antiβ2-glicoprotein I antibodies. As the presence of low-titer anticardiolipin is frequent in subjects with CLD, the diagnostic criteria for APS in such patients requires, apart from past evidence of thrombosis or miscarriages, the detection of one of those antibodies in medium or high titers two times at least 12 weeks apart.[17,37,38]

Inherited deficiencies of antithrombin and proteins S and C are responsible for 15% to 30% of the cases of PVT and BCS. However, their diagnoses are sometimes challenging in patients with liver disease, because low protein levels could be a result of impaired hepatic synthesis and not related to inherited deficiency. In accordance with this assumption is the reversal of coagulation factor abnormalities after surgical treatment of extrahepatic portal vein obstruction (EHPVO) by mesenteric to left portal vein bypass.[39] In practice, deficiency of proteins S and C and antithrombin are assumed when no other abnormality in the coagulation factors levels is disclosed, indicating preserved liver function. Family studies could also be useful in doubtful cases.[13]

Several other divergent situations deserve mention in this section. Increased levels of factor VIII have also been described in patients with BCS and PVT.[2–5] However, as factor VIII is an acute phase protein, its increase could reflect liver disease per se and not inherited thrombophilia. Diagnosis has to rely on the determination of factor VIII levels as well as other acute phase proteins in different time points. Family studies could also be useful in this situation. In contrast, prothrombin G20210A gene mutation and factor V G1691A gene variant are frequently encountered in this setting. Their diagnosis is straightforward based on polymerase chain reaction (PCR)-based assays.[4,5] However, the role of high homocysteine levels in thrombosis is controversial. Hyperhomocysteinemia can be detected by high performance liquid chromatography or chemiluminescence. Testing solely for methylene tetrahydrofolate reductase (MTHFR) C677T gene mutation is unreliable since heterozygosity and homozygosity for MTHFR C677T variant is observed in 50% and 10% of the healthy population, respectively.[4,5] Paroxysmal nocturnal hemoglobinuria and Behcet's disease may also be observed, particularly in subjects with BCS.[2,7,40]

Based on recommendations from an expert panel, the investigation of thrombophilia in patients with BCS and PVT should initially include complete blood cell count, assays for plasma levels of coagulation factors and inhibitors, determination of genetic factor V and prothrombin gene mutations, assessment of antiphospholipid antibodies and lupus anticoagulant, and flow cytometry testing for paroxysmal nocturnal hemoglobinuria. Bone marrow biopsy, determination of blood cell mass and serum erythropoietin, as well as EEC, and the recently discovered JAK2 mutation should be the next steps in the evaluation of MPD (**Table 3**).[2,3,7]

PORTAL VEIN THROMBOSIS

Extrahepatic obstruction of the portal vein can be caused by thrombosis or by compression or occlusion of the portal trunk or one of its branches by tumors, particularly hepatocellular carcinoma.[1,3,41] In autopsy studies, PVT was found in approximately 1% of the cases, most of them related to cirrhosis or liver cancer with less than one third of the cases attributable to noncirrhotic, nonmalignant PVT.[42] To better characterize those patients without malignancy, two recent consensus conferences[1,41] have recommended the term EHPVO to encompass not only the subjects with recent PVT,

Table 3
Approach to the investigation of acquired and/or inherited thrombophilia in patients with BCS and EHPVO

Myeloproliferative disorders	Complete blood cell count
	Bone marrow biopsy
	Determination of total red cell mass and serum erythropoietin after correction for iron deficiency
	EEC and JAK2 mutation (whether available)
Paroxysmal nocturnal hemoglobinuria	Flow cytometry for CD55- and CD59-deficient cells
Antiphospholipid syndrome	Lupus anticoagulant,[a] IgM and IgG anticardiolipin antibodies, antib2-glicoprotein I and antinuclear factors
Factor V Leiden mutation	Detection of G1691A gene variant by PCR-based methods
Prothrombin gene mutation	Detection of G20210A gene mutation by PCR-based methods
Protein C, S, and Antithrombin III	Functional assays in the presence of normal clotting factor levels plasma levels[a]
Hyperhomocysteinemia	Blood folate, vitamin B12 and homocysteine levels. Search for MTHFR polymorphism only when the level of homocysteine is high

Abbreviations: BCS, Budd–Chiari syndrome; EEC, endogenous erythrocyte colonies; EHPVO, extrahepatic portal vein obstruction; JAK2, Janus kinase-2; MTHFR, methylene tetrahydrofolate reductase; PCR, polymerase chain reaction.

[a] Levels are influenced by anticoagulation; testing for multiple abnormalities is advisable, because several patients with BCS and portal vein thrombosis had one or more overlapping prothrombotic risk factors.

but also those with the chronic form known as portal cavernoma. The panel also suggested the categorization as distinct subgroups the cases of intrahepatic PVT and PVT in association with cirrhosis. The following sections address several types of EHPVO beginning with that observed in childhood and concluding with cirrhosis-associated forms of this disorder.

Extrahepatic Portal Vein Obstruction in Childhood

The frequency of EHPVO is higher in Asia and South America, where it affects mainly children. Most of the cases of EHPVO in childhood are either idiopathic[41,43,44] or associated with a past history of umbilical sepsis or umbilical vein catheterization.[45] Even though inherited or acquired thrombophilia were reported to be rare in children with EHPVO,[41,43,44] one Egyptian study has described the association of one or more inherited prothrombotic disorders in up to 63% of the children with EHPVO.[46]

Clinical manifestations in children are mainly a result of portal hypertension.[41,47,48] Most have chronic EHPVO with portal cavernoma disclosed by ultrasound (US) or by MRI or CT angiogram. Variceal bleeding is the most common presentation, but cholestasis caused by portal biliopathy (biliary abnormalities including strictures as a result of extrinsic bile duct compression by dilated venous collaterals), growth retardation, and abdominal distension as a result of splenomegaly or pancytopenia caused by hypersplenism may also occur at presentation. The natural history of EHPVO is usually benign. However, some patients may develop signs of liver failure, which may be ascribed to concurrent hepatitis B or C or liver dysfunction as a result of parenchymal extinction.[49] Management of EHPVO in children is based on uncontrolled studies and includes sclerotherapy or endoscopic band ligation (EBL) for the control of acute variceal bleeding and EBL and/or beta-blockers for secondary prophylaxis.

Anticoagulation should be restricted to those subjects with recognizable prothrombotic disorders. Portal biliopathy treatment is advised only for symptomatic cases, preferably by endoscopic therapy.[41] Surgical shunts, particularly distal splenorenal shunts, have been performed for variceal bleeding or portal biliopathy refractory to endoscopic therapy, but the use of mesenteric to left portal vein bypass (Rex shunt) has been advocated to be more physiologic, as it restores portal venous blood flow to the liver via the left portal vein in the Rex recessus.[50,51] The use of Rex shunts has been associated with excellent long-term outcomes including no further bleeding episodes from varices, partial or complete regression of splenomegaly, improvement in platelet and leukocyte counts, and normalization of coagulation abnormalities in most of the surgically treated subjects.[39] These findings altogether have led some authorities to consider this surgical procedure as the therapy of choice for symptomatic EHPVO in children, when technically feasible.[51]

Nonmalignant, Noncirrhotic Extrahepatic Portal Vein Obstruction in Adults

Nontumoral EHPVO in adults can be classified according to presentation as acute PVT or chronic EHPVO, as well as to the presence or absence of cirrhosis, which is discussed separately in the next section.[3] Portal vein thrombosis can also occur in association with other liver diseases caused by prothrombotic disorders such as BCS or noncirrhotic portal hypertension (NCPH).[52] In adults, noncirrhotic, nontumoral EHPVO is quite rare and accounts for less than 10% of the cases of portal hypertension with fewer than 400 patients reported from three reference centers in Europe.[3,8,9,53]

Clinical findings and management options vary according to the type of EHPVO. Acute or recent PVT is characterized by recent occlusion of the portal vein by a thrombus that can be associated or not with symptoms of abdominal pain and diarrhea, as well as signs of systemic inflammatory response or sepsis in case of pylephlebitis.[3] Severity depends on the extent of involvement of the portal venous system. Bloody diarrhea, ascites, and ileus are more common in severe superior mesenteric vein involvement that may lead to mesenteric ischemia with bowel perforation and septic shock. The diagnosis is usually performed by US, which shows hyperechoic material in the portal vein with downstream dilatation of the portal venous system with no flow detected by Doppler imaging (**Fig. 1**).

Chronic EHPVO is the late-stage sequela of PVT usually defined by the presence of portal cavernoma, characterized by replacement of the portal vein by fibrous tissue and development of periportal collateral vessels bypassing the obstructed portal vein segment.[3,41] Chronic EHPVO leads to portal hypertension with a higher frequency of bleeding from ectopic varices when compared with cirrhosis.[41] Other less frequent manifestations of chronic EHPVO include portal cholangiopathy and hepatic encephalopathy.[3,41,54] Portal cholangiopathy is caused by encasement of bile ducts by dilated peribiliar collaterals leading to irregularities and strictures of the biliary tree particularly at the hilum. These abnormalities may be similar to those observed in primary sclerosing cholangitis and have been reported in up to 80% to 100% of the patients adequately examined by endoscopic retrograde cholangiopancreatography (ERCP) or by magnetic resonance cholangiopancreatography (MRCP). Signs and symptoms of cholestasis or cholangitis are nevertheless quite uncommon. Overt hepatic encephalopathy is rare and is due to the presence of large shunts, but minimal hepatic encephalopathy has been reported in 50% of the patients with chronic EHPVO when assessed by neuropsychological tests, brain MRI imaging, or the oral glutamine

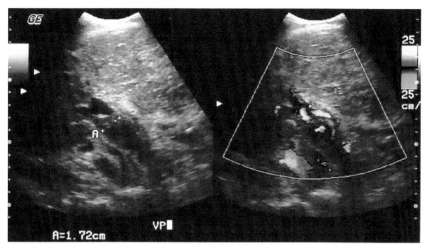

Fig. 1. Doppler ultrasound showing echogenic material in the portal vein with downstream dilatation of the portal venous system and no flow detected by Doppler imaging. (*Courtesy of* Magid Abud, MD, Salvador, Bahia, Brazil.)

challenge test.[54] Diagnosis of chronic EHPVO is usually made by imaging with US and MRI or CT (**Fig. 2**).

The natural history of acute and chronic EHPVO in adults is often relatively benign. Survival is frequently more related to the presence or absence of an associated disorder. In the absence of cirrhosis, massive superior mesenteric vein thrombosis, and

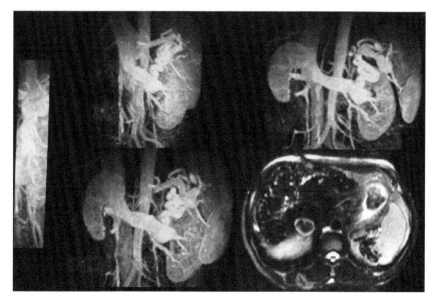

Fig. 2. MR angiography in a patient with cavernous transformation of portal vein. Esophageal varices (on the left): no delineation of the portal vein, enlargement of the splenic vein, and left renal vein because of the presence of a large spontaneous splenorenal shunt. (*Courtesy of* Helio Braga, MD, Salvador, Bahia, Brazil.)

cancer, a survival rate of 81% at 10 years has been reported.[53] Mortality is usually related to associated clinical disorders, recurrent thrombotic events, or to the occurrence of massive variceal bleeding.

Because of their rarity, most of the management options and treatment strategies for acute and chronic EHPVO are not based on strong scientific evidence. Guidelines endorsed by the Asian Pacific Association for the Study of the Liver and the Baveno IV Consensus Workshop have been recently published addressing recommendations regarding the current knowledge on acute and chronic EHPVO.[1,41] Management of acute or recent PVT includes treatment of associated infectious or inflammatory disorders and therapy directed toward recanalization of the portal vein, prevention of thrombus extension into the superior mesenteric veins, as well as recurrent thrombosis in those subjects with recognizable prothrombotic risk factors. Based on retrospective analysis of selected cohorts of patients,[55,56] anticoagulation has been recommended in acute PVT for at least 3 months, with the suggestion that it may be lifelong in those subjects with prothrombotic disorders.[1,41] This strategy has been associated with high rates of recanalization of the portal vein with few bleeding events and no mortality as well as no progression to cavernoma and portal hypertension attributable to chronic EHPVO. Recently, one multicentric prospective study involving 105 patients has shown a recanalization rate of 44% at 1 year after anticoagulation, which was higher in subjects with recent PVT without ascites. No recurrence of splanchnic vein thrombosis was reported and mortality was 2%.[57]

Several surgical and interventional procedures, including mechanical thrombectomy, systemic or percutaneous transcatheter thrombolysis, angioplasty, or transjugular intrahepatic portosystemic shunt (TIPS), have been performed in subjects with PVT.[58,59] These techniques were shown to be feasible when performed at referral centers and efficacious in selected patients, but major adverse events have been reported in up to 60% of the patients treated by interventional radiology.[58] The Asian consensus has considered percutaneous transhepatic permeation of the portal vein only in patients with progressive recent EHPVO with signs of ongoing mesenteric ischemia despite anticoagulation.[41]

There are no evidence-based data regarding the role of anticoagulation for chronic EHPVO; however, both consensus documents recommend it for patients with known prothrombotic disorders because of the risk of thrombosis recurrence. One retrospective study from France reported long-term results of anticoagulation for 84 subjects with chronic EHPVO. Bleeding events were related to large varices at admission and severity of bleeding was similar in patients with and without anticoagulation. Thrombotic events were related to the presence of thrombophilia or absence of anticoagulation. Mortality was 7% and was not related to anticoagulation.[56] Management of portal hypertension in subjects with chronic EHPVO is less clear when compared with cirrhotic patients because of the lack of controlled data. There is no consensus regarding the best strategy for primary prophylaxis of variceal bleeding. Regarding the control of acute bleeding episodes, endoscopic therapy is recommended with no data on the use of pharmacologic therapy. For secondary prophylaxis, endoscopic therapy is effective, but there are no data on beta-blockers.[1,41] Portal biliopathy with dominant strictures should be treated when symptomatic with therapeutic endoscopy. Shunt surgery is advised in case of endoscopic failure.[1,41]

Portal Vein Thrombosis in Chronic Liver Disease

The prevalence of EHPVO in cirrhosis is estimated at 1%, increasing in accordance with disease progression to 8% to 15% of the patients with Child B or C CLD.[60,61] Symptoms are observed in half of them, either variceal bleeding or abdominal pain with or without mesenteric ischemia. Apart from advanced liver disease, other risk factors recognized for PVT in cirrhotic patients were male sex, previous treatment for portal hypertension, splenomegaly, and alcoholic liver disease, as well as the presence of inherited prothrombotic disorders, particularly factor II G20210A mutation.[60,62]

The frequency of PVT was also reported to rise in patients on the waiting list for orthotopic liver transplantation (OLT) from 8% at admission to 15% at the time of OLT.[61] In this regard, the occurrence of PVT has been associated with higher incidence of postoperative complications and mortality after OLT, particularly in those subjects with complete occlusion of the portal vein with or without involvement of the superior mesenteric vein.[61,63] Based on these findings, Francoz and colleagues[61] from the Beaujon group have attempted to institute anticoagulation to patients with PVT on the waiting list for OLT. They have described partial or complete recanalization in 42% of the treated subjects with no major adverse event reported.

BUDD–CHIARI SYNDROME

Budd–Chiari syndrome is an uncommon and heterogeneous group of disorders characterized by hepatic venous outflow obstruction at any level from the small hepatic veins to the junction of the IVC and the right atrium.[7,64] By definition, outflow obstruction because of heart failure or veno-occlusive disease secondary to nonthrombotic obstruction of the hepatic microcirculation are not considered as variants of BCS.[7]

The prevalence of BCS is estimated as 1:100,000, with fewer than 300 patients reported from three tertiary referral centers in the Netherlands, France, and the United States.[65,66] Obstruction of the hepatic venous outflow tract is classified according to its anatomic impairment, as at the small hepatic veins, large hepatic veins, or IVC (**Table 4**). Obstruction can occur at more than one of these sites, particularly involving the large hepatic veins and IVC.[7] Obstruction of the IVC is more common in the East and is associated with increased frequency of hepatocellular carcinoma.[2] In the West, it is more often found in subjects with factor V Leiden mutation or Behcet's disease. On the other hand, isolated involvement of small hepatic veins is more commonly observed in subjects with paroxysmal nocturnal hemoglobinuria.[2]

It can also be classified as primary when the obstruction results from an endoluminal thrombus or by thrombosis-associated webs, which are now recognized as late-stage sequelae of thrombosis,[21,61] or as secondary when there is an extrinsic invasion or compression of the hepatic veins or IVC by tumors or non-neoplastic mass-forming lesions such as cysts or abscesses (**Table 5**).[7,67] For practical purposes, BCS is considered as primary when no extrinsic causes of secondary obstruction are found by current imaging techniques. Several other classifications based on clinical disease severity or duration such as acute, subacute, and chronic BCS or fulminant BCS have been proposed based on putative differences in prognosis and management.[68–72] However, these classifications are recommended only for descriptive purposes, as they have not been validated in prospective studies and also have not been endorsed because of the lack of well-established criteria for their definition.[7]

The clinical course of BCS can vary markedly, ranging from asymptomatic disease to fulminant liver failure,[68–72] depending on the speed of occlusion, the extent of hepatic vein involvement, and on whether a venous collateral circulation has developed to decompress the liver sinusoids. Most patients present painful hepatomegaly and ascites.[70–72] Differential diagnosis with sinusoidal obstruction syndrome (SOS) and cardiac insufficiency is important, as these entities may present with similar clinical features.[7] Heart failure can be ruled out by careful physical examination and echocardiography when appropriate. SOS, formerly known as veno-occlusive disease,[2,73]

Table 4
Classification of Budd–Chiari syndrome according to site of obstruction

Site of Obstruction	Frequency According to Imaging Techniques	Criteria
Small hepatic veins	NA	Involvement of veins that cannot be clearly shown on hepatic venograms or ultrasound, including terminal hepatic veins, and intercalated and interlobular veins
Large hepatic veins[a]	50%	Involvement of veins that are regularly seen on hepatic venograms and ultrasound, including segmental branches of hepatic veins
Inferior vena cava (IVC)	2%	Involvement of one segment of the IVC, which extends from the entry level of the right, middle, and left hepatic veins to the junction between the IVC and the right atrium
Combined obstruction	47%	Involvement of the large hepatic veins and IVC

Abbreviation: NA, not applicable.
[a] Pure hepatic vein involvement is more frequent in Western when compared with Eastern countries.[65]
Data from Janssen HL, Garcia-Pagan JC, Elias E, et al. Budd–Chiari syndrome: a review by an expert panel. J Hepatol 2003;38:364–71; and Plessier A, Denninger MH, Casadevall N, et al. Relevance of the criteria commonly used to diagnose myeloproliferative disorder in patients with splanchnic vein thrombosis. Br J Haematol 2005;129:553–60.

usually occurs after myeloablative hematopoietic stem cell transplantation, when its diagnosis is usually straightforward. However, when SOS is associated with ingestion of pyrrolizidine alkaloids or other drugs, liver biopsy is usually required for its diagnosis.

According to recommendations from an expert panel report,[7] BCS should be suspected in patients with abrupt onset of ascites and painful hepatomegaly, massive ascites without major impairment in liver function, fulminant hepatic failure associated with hepatomegaly and ascites, or liver disease associated with inherited or acquired thrombophilia, as well as in subjects with unexplained chronic liver disease. Ascites

Table 5
Classification of Budd–Chiari syndrome according to etiology

Etiology	Criteria
Primary	Hepatic venous outflow obstruction resulting from endoluminal venous lesion (thrombosis, webs, endophlebitis). Of note, webs are now recognized as late-stage sequel of thrombosis.
Secondary	Hepatic venous outflow obstruction caused by invasion or obstruction from a lesion outside the hepatic outflow venous system (tumor, abscess, cysts).

Adapted from Janssen HL, Garcia-Pagan JC, Elias E, et al. Budd–Chiari syndrome: a review by an expert panel. J Hepatol 2003;38:364–71; with permission.

fluid analysis, which typically shows high protein, high albumin gradient in the absence of heart failure can also be a practical clue to the presence of BCS. The diagnosis is usually established by Doppler ultrasonography (DU), which demonstrates thrombosis or absence of hepatic veins; absent, reversed, or turbulent flow; or occurrence of collateral hepatic venous circulation, as well as enlargement of the caudate lobe. Sensitivity and specificity for DU ranges from 75% to 85%.[72,74] Nonvisualized or tortuous hepatic veins are common but nonspecific sonographic findings of BCS, while intrahepatic or subcapsular venous collaterals are sensitive sonographic findings (**Fig. 3**).[72,74–76] CT is superior to DU to assess IVC involvement and to reveal liver perfusion defects (**Fig. 4**).[74]

MRI has been recommended as the second method of investigation (**Fig. 5**),[7] as it allows better delineation of the vascular anatomy of splanchnic vessels without use of contrast agents and is also able to better differentiate acute from chronic BCS.[67,76] Venography is usually performed when noninvasive imaging techniques fail to provide clear-cut diagnosis of BCS in patients with a high index of suspicion of the disease or when surgical shunts are a treatment option to assess the occurrence of IVC obstruction by pressure measurements. Liver biopsy is rarely used for diagnostic purposes but it has been recently used for prognosis.[77] In this regard, the presence of acute injuries associated with chronic lesions on liver biopsy has been associated with shortened survival.[77]

Prognosis has been improved markedly in recent years, with survival rates of 77% to 82%, 65% to 69%, and 57% to 62%, at 1, 5, and 10 years, respectively,[65,78,79]

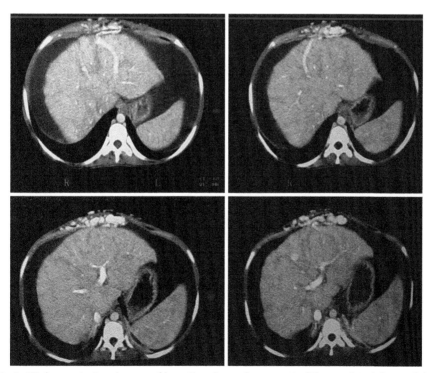

Fig. 3. CT demonstrates absence of hepatic veins, enlargement of the caudate lobe, and the presence of intrahepatic and subcapsular venous collaterals. (*Courtesy of* Luciana Costa Silva, MD, PhD, Minas Gerais, Brazil.)

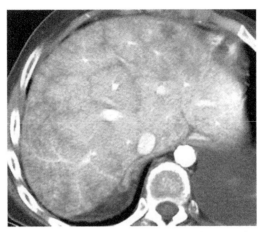

Fig. 4. CT scanning showing diffuse perfusion defects and absence of the hepatic veins.

probably because of improved recognition of BCS, particularly asymptomatic cases, and more frequent use of anticoagulation.[2,78] The risk of death is highest within the first 1 to 2 years after diagnosis, whereas patients surviving beyond 2 years have excellent long-term survival rates.[37–39] Adverse outcomes have been associated with age at presentation, poor response of ascitis to diuretics, Child-Pugh score, and renal failure,[78] as well as the occurrence of encephalopathy, ascitis, enlarged prothrombin time, and hyperbilirrubinemia.[65]

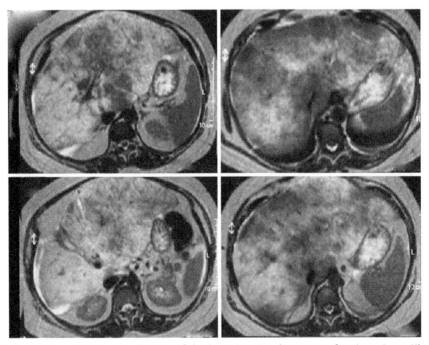

Fig. 5. MRI in a patient with absence of the hepatic veins. (*Courtesy of* Luciana Costa Silva, MD, PhD, Minas Gerais, Brazil.)

Strategies for the treatment of BCS are not evidence-based because of the rarity of this disorder and the lack of randomized controlled trials evaluating current available treatment options, including medical management aimed at control of underlying diseases and complications of portal hypertension, as well as anticoagulation and surgical treatment with portosystemic shunts (PSS) or OLT and interventional radiology with angioplasty coupled or not with thrombolysis and TIPS.[80] Two expert opinion reports have been published regarding the management of BCS.[1,7]

Management of ascitis and prevention and treatment of portal hypertensive bleeding in patients with BCS are not different when compared with cirrhotic patients and subjects with EHPVO,[1] but data concerning treatment issues in BCS are scanty even when compared with EHPVO. Anticoagulation is recommended in the presence of recent or long-standing thrombosis to allow recanalization or to avoid thrombus progression or recurrence. Surgical or radiological approaches to relieve sinusoidal pressure in patients with BCS have been advocated,[80] but they were not associated with improvement in survival[65,78] and are now considered appropriate only for symptomatic patients who do not improve with medical management.[1,2,7] Interventional radiology using percutaneous thrombolysis and angioplasty with or without stenting could be a first-line strategy for selected patients with recent thrombosis or subjects with short-length stenosis of the IVC or hepatic veins with excellent outcomes reported from centers with skillful radiology teams.[19,81]

Use of PSS was advocated as a definite measure to relieve sinusoidal hypertension with the potential to reverse hepatic necrosis and prevent cirrhosis. It is now largely replaced by TIPS. However, both treatment modalities have been associated with high rates of shunt dysfunction, requiring revision and leading to increased morbidity.[2,81,82] Liver transplantation is required when the aforementioned treatment strategies fail in patients with a progressive downhill course with 1-, 5-, and 10-year survival rates of 76%, 71%, and 68%, respectively.[82] Renal failure and presence of PSS and/or TIPS before OLT were associated with shortened survival. Anticoagulation is required after OLT to prevent recurrence of thrombosis, which may occur in 2% to 27% of the cases.[82,83]

ASSOCIATION OF BUDD–CHIARI SYNDROME, EXTRAHEPATIC PORTAL VEIN OBSTRUCTION, AND NONCIRRHOTIC PORTAL HYPERTENSION

Extrahepatic portal vein obstruction may overlap with other vascular disorders of the liver, particularly with BCS and NCPH. In a multicenter European cohort of BCS, EHPVO was observed in 18% of the affected subjects.[52] The clinical presentation was similar irrespective of the presence of EHPVO, however two or more prothrombotic risk factors tended to be more frequent in patients with associated splanchnic vein thrombosis. Survival also tended to be reduced in subjects with BCS-associated EHPVO. Hepatoportal sclerosis is another vascular disorder of the liver that is frequent in the East and leads to NCPH.[41,84] Thrombosis of the medium to small portal veins has been recently linked to its pathogenesis.[41] In a retrospective review of 28 Western patients followed for 7.6 years, EHPVO was shown to develop in 46% of the cases.[85] Most of those subjects had associated prothrombotic disorders, particularly chronic MPD.

SUMMARY

Nonmalignant, noncirrhotic EHPVO and Budd–Chiari syndrome are mainly caused by several heterogeneous inherited and acquired prothrombotic disorders. Investigation of thrombophilia can be difficult in this setting and a formal hematological consultation is usually required. Variceal bleeding caused by portal hypertension is the most frequent clinical manifestation of EHPVO, but cholestasis caused by portal biliopathy, growth retardation, splenomegaly, and pancytopenia caused by hypersplenism and hepatic encephalopathy may also occur. Treatment options are based on uncontrolled data and include anticoagulation to prevent thrombosis extension or recurrence and prophylaxis as well as treatment of complications of portal hypertension. In children, excellent long-term outcomes have been reported with the use of mesenteric to left portal vein bypass (Rex shunt). The natural history of nonmalignant, noncirrhotic EHPVO in adults is relatively benign and survival is directly related to the presence of an associated prothrombotic disorder.

The clinical course of BCS can vary from asymptomatic disease to fulminant liver failure, depending on the speed and the extent of the occlusion. Most patients present with painful hepatomegaly and high-protein fluid ascites. Doppler ultrasonography is usually required for diagnosis. Prognosis has improved markedly in recent years, but age at presentation; poor response of ascites to diuretics; Child-Pugh score; and the occurrence of renal failure, hepatic encephalopathy, increased prothrombin time, and hyperbilirrubinemia have been associated with adverse outcomes. Strategies for the treatment of BCS are not evidence-based and should be individualized. Medical management includes anticoagulation for those subjects with prothrombotic risk factors and control of the complications of portal hypertension, such as ascites and variceal bleeding. Other treatment options include surgical portosystemic shunts, TIPS, or liver transplantation. Recently, medical management has been favored as first-line therapy, because surgical and radiological approaches to relieve sinusoidal pressure in patients with BCS have not been shown to improve survival. In patients with failure of medical therapy and a progressive downhill course, TIPS and liver transplantation are advocated with excellent long-term survival.

REFERENCES

1. De Franchis R. Evolving consensus in portal hypertension. Report of the Baveno IV consensus workshop on methodology of diagnosis and therapy in portal hypertension. J Hepatol 2005;43:167–76.
2. Valla DC. The diagnosis and management of the Budd–Chiari syndrome: consensus and controversies. Hepatology 2003;38:793–803.
3. Condat B, Valla D. Nonmalignant portal vein thrombosis in adults. Nat Clin Pract Gastroenterol Hepatol 2006;3:505–15.
4. Middeldorp S, Levi M. Thrombophilia: an update. Semin Thromb Hemost 2007; 33:563–72.
5. Simioni P, Tormene D, Spiezia L, et al. Inherited thrombophilia and venous thromboembolism. Semin Thromb Hemost 2006;32:700–8.
6. Franco RF, Trip MP, Reitsma PH. Genetic variations of the hemostatic system as a risk factor for venous and arterial thrombotic disease. Curr Genomics 2003;4: 1–21.
7. Janssen HL, Garcia-Pagan JC, Elias E, et al. Budd–Chiari syndrome: a review by an expert panel. J Hepatol 2003;38:364–71.
8. Primignani M, Martinelli I, Bucciarelli P, et al. Risk factors for thrombophilia in extrahepatic portal vein obstruction. Hepatology 2005;41:603–8.
9. Denninger MH, Chait Y, Casadevall N, et al. Cause of portal or hepatic venous thrombosis in adults: the role of multiple concurrent factors. Hepatology 2000; 31:587–91.

10. Janssen HL, Meinardi JR, Vleggaar FP, et al. Factor V Leiden mutation, prothrombin gene mutation, and deficiencies in coagulation inhibitors associated with Budd–Chiari syndrome and portal vein thrombosis: results of a case-control study. Blood 2000;96:2364–8.
11. Bhattacharyya M, Makharia G, Kannan M, et al. Inherited prothrombotic defects in Budd–Chiari syndrome and portal vein thrombosis: a study from North India. Am J Clin Pathol 2004;121:844–7.
12. Mohanty D, Shetty S, Ghosh K, et al. Hereditary thrombophilia as a cause of Budd–Chiari syndrome: a study from western India. Hepatology 2001;34: 666–70.
13. Brie JB. Budd–Chiari syndrome and portal vein thrombosis associated with myeloproliferative disorders: diagnosis and management. Semin Thromb Hemost 2006;32:208–18.
14. Deltenre P, Denninger MH, Hillaire S, et al. Factor V Leiden related Budd–Chiari syndrome. Gut 2001;48:264–8.
15. Aydinli M, Bayraktar Y. Budd–Chiari syndrome: etiology, pathogenesis and diagnosis. World J Gastroenterol 2007;13:2693–6.
16. Li XM, Wei YF, Hao HL, et al. Hyperhomocysteinemia and the MTHFR C677T mutation in Budd–Chiari syndrome. Am J Hematol 2002;71:11–4.
17. Lim W, Crowther MA. Antiphospholipid antibodies: a critical review of the literature. Curr Opin Hematol 2007;14:494–9.
18. Cohn DM, Roshani S, Middeldorp S. Thrombophilia and venous thromboembolism: implications for testing. Semin Thromb Hemost 2007;33:573–81.
19. Sharma S, Kumar SI, Poddar U, et al. Factor V Leiden and prothrombin gene G20210A mutations are uncommon in portal vein thrombosis in India. Indian J Gastroenterol 2006;25:236–9.
20. Valla DC. Portal vein thrombosis and prothrombotic disorders. J Gastroenterol Hepatol 1999;14:1051–2.
21. Valla DC. Hepatic venous outflow tract obstruction etiopathogenesis: Asia versus the West. J Gastroenterol Hepatol 2004;19:S204–11.
22. Heit JA. Thrombophilia: common questions on laboratory assessment and management. Educational Book. Hematology 2007;127–35.
23. Chait Y, Condat B, Cazals-Hatem D, et al. Relevance of the criteria commonly used to diagnose myeloproliferative disorder in patients with splanchnic vein thrombosis. Br J Haematol 2005;129:553–60.
24. Patel RK, Nicholas CL, Heneghan MA, et al. Prevalence of the activating *JAK2* tyrosine kinase mutation V617F in the Budd–Chiari syndrome. Gastroenterology 2006;130:2031–8.
25. Thurmes PJ, Steensma DP. Elevated serum erythropoietin levels in patients with Budd–Chiari syndrome secondary to polycythemia vera: clinical implications for the role of JAK2 mutation analysis. Eur J Haematol 2006;77:57–60.
26. Colaizzo D, Amitrano L, Tiscia GL, et al. The JAK2 V617F mutation frequently occurs in patients with portal and mesenteric venous thrombosis. J Thromb Haemost 2007;5:55–61.
27. Jones AV, Kreil S, Zoi K, et al. Widespread occurrence of the *JAK2* V617F mutation in chronic myeloproliferative disorders. Blood 2005;106:2162–8.
28. De Stefano V, Fiorini A, Rossi E, et al. Incidence of the JAK2 V617F mutation among patients with splanchnic or cerebral venous thrombosis and without overt chronic myeloproliferative disorders. J Thromb Haemost 2007;5:708–14.
29. Kaushansky K. On the molecular origins of the chronic myeloproliferative disorders: it all makes sense. Blood 2005;105:4258–63.

30. Dudley JM, Westwood N, Leonard S, et al. Primary polycythemia: positive diagnosis using the differential response of primitive and mature erythroid progenitors to erythropoietin, interleukin 3 and alpha-interferon. Br J Haematol 1990;75:188–94.

31. Dainiak N, Hoffman R, Lebowitz AI, et al. Erythropoietin-dependent primary pure erythrocytosis. Blood 1979;53:1076–84.

32. Eridani S, Dudley JM, Sawyer BM, et al. Erythropoietic colonies in a serum-free system: results in primary proliferative polycythemia and thrombocythemias. Br J Haematol 1987;67:387–91.

33. Levine RL, Wernig G. Role of JAK-STAT signaling in the pathogenesis of myeloproliferative disorders. Hematology Am Soc Hematol Educ Program 2006;510:233–9.

34. Kralovics R, Passamonti F, Buser AS, et al. A gain-of-function mutation of JAK2 in myeloproliferative disorders. N Engl J Med 2005;352:1779–90.

35. Kiladjian JJ, Cervantes F, Leebeek FW, et al. The impact of JAK2 and MPL mutations on diagnosis and prognosis of splanchnic vein thrombosis: a report on 241 cases. Blood 2008;111:4922–9.

36. Murad SD, Plessier A, Hernandez Guerra M, et al. A prospective follow-up study on 163 patients with Budd–Chiari syndrome: results from the European network for vascular disorders of the liver (EM_VIE). J Hepatol 2007;46:S4 [abstract].

37. Levine JS, Branch DW, Rauch J. The antiphospholipid syndrome. N Engl J Med 2002;346:752–63.

38. Miyakis S, Lockshin MD, Atsumi T, et al. International consensus statement on an update of the classification criteria for definite antiphospholipid syndrome (APS). J Thromb Haemost 2006;4:296–306.

39. Superina R, Bambini DA, Lokar J, et al. Correction of extrahepatic portal vein thrombosis by the mesenteric to left portal vein bypass. Ann Surg 2006;243:515–21.

40. Ziakas PD, Poulou LS, Rokas GI, et al. Thrombosis in paroxysmal nocturnal hemoglobinuria: sites, risks, outcome. An overview. J Thromb Haemost 2007;5:642–5.

41. Sarin SK, Sollano JD, Chawla YK, et al. Consensus on extra-hepatic portal vein obstruction. Liver Int 2006;26:512–9.

42. Ogren M, Bergqvist D, Bjorck M, et al. Portal vein thrombosis: prevalence, patient characteristics and lifetime risk: a population study based on 23,796 consecutive autopsies. World J Gastroenterol 2006;12:2115–9.

43. Pinto RB, Silveira TR, Bandinelli E, et al. Portal vein thrombosis in children and adolescents: the low prevalence of hereditary thrombophilic disorders. J Pediatr Surg 2004;39:1356–61.

44. Pugliese RPS, Porta G, D'Amico EA, et al. Risk factors in children and adolescents with portal vein thrombosis (PVT) and portal hypertension. Hepatology 1998;28:551A.

45. Alvarez F. Risk of portal obstruction in newborns. J Pediatr 2006;148:715–6.

46. El-Karaksy H, El-Koofy N, El-Hawary M, et al. Prevalence of factor V Leiden mutation and other hereditary thrombophilic factors in Egyptian children with portal vein thrombosis: results of a single-center case-control study. Ann Hematol 2004;83:712–5.

47. Lykavieris P, Gauthier F, Hadchouel P, et al. Risk of gastrointestinal bleeding during adolescence and early adulthood in children with portal vein obstruction. J Pediatr 2000;136:805–8.

48. Alvarez F, Bernard O, Brunelle F, et al. Portal obstruction in children. I. Clinical investigation and hemorrhage risk. J Pediat 1983;103:696–702.

49. Rangari M, Gupta R, Jain M, et al. Hepatic dysfunction in patients with extrahepatic portal venous obstruction. Liver Int 2003;23:434–9.
50. De Ville de Goyet J, Gibbs P, Clapuyt P, et al. Original extrahilar approach for hepatic portal revascularization and relief of extrahepatic portal hypertension related to later portal vein thrombosis after pediatric liver transplantation. Long-term results. Transplantation 1996;62:71–5.
51. Superina R, Shneider B, Emre S, et al. Surgical guidelines for the management of extra-hepatic portal vein obstruction. Pediatr Transplant 2006;10:908–13.
52. Murad SD, Valla DC, de Groen PC, et al. Pathogenesis and treatment of Budd–Chiari syndrome combined with portal vein thrombosis. Am J Gastroenterol 2006;101:83–90.
53. Janssen HL, Wijnhoud A, Haagsma EB, et al. Extrahepatic portal vein thrombosis: aetiology and determinants of survival. Gut 2001;49:720–4.
54. Mínguez B, García-Pagán JC, Bosch J, et al. Noncirrhotic portal vein thrombosis exhibits neuropsychological and MR changes consistent with minimal hepatic encephalopathy. Hepatology 2006;43:707–14.
55. Condat B, Pessione F, Hillaire S, et al. Recent portal or mesenteric venous thrombosis: increased recognition and frequent recanalization on anticoagulant therapy. Hepatology 2000;32:466–70.
56. Condat B, Pessione F, Hillaire S, et al. Current outcome of portal vein thrombosis in adults: risk and benefit of anticoagulant therapy. Gastroenterology 2001;120:490–7.
57. Plessier A, Murad SD, Hernandez Guerra M, et al. A prospective multicentric follow-up study on 105 patients with acute portal vein thrombosis (PVT): results from the European network for vascular disorders of the liver (EM-VIE). Hepatology 2007;46:309A [abstract].
58. Hollingshead M, Burke CT, Mauro MA, et al. Transcatheter thrombolytic therapy for acute mesenteric and portal vein thrombosis. J Vasc Interv Radiol 2005;16:651–61.
59. Senzolo M, Tibbals J, Cholongitas E, et al. Transjugular intrahepatic portosystemic shunt for portal vein thrombosis with and without cavernous transformation. Aliment Pharmacol Ther 2006;23:767–75.
60. Amitrano L, Guardascione MA, Brancaccio V, et al. Risk factors and clinical presentation of portal vein thrombosis in patients with liver cirrhosis. J Hepatol 2004;40:736–41.
61. Francoz C, Belghiti J, Vilgrain V, et al. Splanchnic vein thrombosis in candidates for liver transplantation: usefulness of screening and anticoagulation. Gut 2006;54:691–7.
62. Amitrano L, Brancaccio V, Guardascione MA, et al. Inherited coagulation disorders in cirrhotic patients with portal vein thrombosis. Hepatology 2000;31:345–8.
63. Yerdel MA, Gunson B, Mirza D, et al. Portal vein thrombosis in adults undergoing liver transplantation: risk factors, screening, management, and outcome. Transplantation 2000;69:1873–81.
64. Ludwig J, Hashimoto E, McGill DB, et al. Classification of hepatic venous outflow obstruction: ambiguous terminology of the Budd–Chiari syndrome. Mayo Clin Proc 1990;65:51–5.
65. Murad SD, Valla DC, de Groen PC, et al. Determinants of survival and the effect of portosystemic shunting in patients with Budd–Chiari syndrome. Hepatology 2004;39:500–8.
66. Okuda K. Membranous obstruction of the inferior vena cava (obliterative hepatocavopathy, Okuda). J Gastroenterol Hepatol 2001;16:1179–83.

67. Zimmerman MA, Cameron AM, Ghobrial RM. Budd–Chiari syndrome. Clin Liver Dis 2006;10:259–73.
68. Menon KVN, Shah V, Kamath PS. Current concepts: the Budd–Chiari Syndrome. N Engl J Med 2004;350:578–85.
69. Hadengue A, Poliquin M, Vilgrain V, et al. The changing scene of hepatic vein thrombosis: recognition of asymptomatic cases. Gastroenterology 1994;106: 1042–7.
70. Dilawari JB, Bambery P, Chawla Y, et al. Hepatic outflow obstruction (Budd–Chiari syndrome). Experience with 177 patients and a review of the literature. Medicine (Baltimore) 1994;73:21–36.
71. Mahmoud AE, Mendoza A, Meshikhes AN, et al. Clinical spectrum, investigations and treatment of Budd–Chiari syndrome. Q J Med 1996;89:37–43.
72. Bolondi L, Gaiani S, Li Bassi S, et al. Diagnosis of Budd–Chiari syndrome by pulsed Doppler ultrasound. Gastroenterology 1991;100:1324–31.
73. DeLeve LD, Shulman HM, McDonald GB. Toxic injury to hepatic sinusoids: sinusoidal obstruction syndrome (veno-occlusive disease). Semin Liver Dis 2002;22: 27–42.
74. Kamath P. Budd–Chiari syndrome: radiologic findings. Liver Transp 2006;12: S21–2.
75. Chawla Y, Kumar S, Dhiman RK, et al. Duplex Doppler sonography in patients with Budd–Chiari syndrome. J Gastroenterol Hepatol 1999;14:904–7.
76. Brancatelli G, Vilgrain V, Federle MP, et al. Budd–Chiari syndrome: spectrum of imaging findings. AJR Am J Roentgenol 2007;188(2):168–76.
77. Langlet P, Escolano S, Valla D, et al. Clinicopathological forms and prognostic index in Budd–Chiari syndrome. J Hepatol 2003;39:496–501.
78. Zeitoun G, Escolano S, Hadengue A, et al. Outcome of Budd–Chiari syndrome: a multivariate analysis of factors related to survival including surgical portosystemic shunting. Hepatology 1999;30:84–9.
79. Orloff MJ, Daily PO, Orloff SL, et al. A 27-year experience with surgical treatment of Budd–Chiari syndrome. Ann Surg 2000;232:340–52.
80. Klein AS. Management of Budd–Chiari syndrome. Liver Transpl 2006;12:S23–8.
81. Eapen CE, Velissaris D, Heydtmann M, et al. Favourable medium term outcome following hepatic vein recanalisation and/or transjugular intrahepatic portosystemic shunt for Budd Chiari syndrome. Gut 2006;55:878–84.
82. Mentha G, Giostra E, Majno PE, et al. Liver transplantation for Budd-Chiari syndrome: a European study on 248 patients from 51 centres. J Hepatol 2006; 44:520–8.
83. Cruz E, Ascher NL, Roberts JP, et al. High incidence of recurrence and hematologic events following liver transplantation for Budd-Chiari syndrome. Clin Transplant 2005;19:501–6.
84. Sarin SK, Kumar A. Non-cirrhotic portal hypertension. Clin Liver Dis 2006;10:627–51.
85. Hillaire S, Bonte E, Denninger M-H, et al. Idiopathic non-cirrhotic intrahepatic portal hypertension in the west: a re-evaluation in 28 patients. Gut 2002;51: 275–80.

Bleeding in Liver Surgery: Prevention and Treatment

Edris M. Alkozai, BSc, Ton Lisman, PhD, Robert J. Porte, MD, PhD*

KEYWORDS

- Blood loss • Liver transplantation • Liver resection
- Surgical methods • Central venous pressure • Fibrin sealants
- Aprotinin • Tranexamic acid

Bleeding in major surgical procedures involving the liver, such as partial liver resection and liver transplantation, occurs almost inevitably. Although blood loss in patients undergoing liver surgery has decreased substantially during the last decade, excessive blood loss can still be a major concern in individual patients. Bleeding problems are not limited to surgical patients who have a cirrhotic liver; they may also occur in patients who have a normal liver. Extensive bleeding may require the transfusion of blood or blood products, which are associated with increased rates of morbidity and mortality.[1–6] Although the mechanism of bleeding in surgical interventions is multifactorial, technical factors may be responsible for a significant amount of intraoperative and early postoperative bleeding.[7] Besides surgical factors, abnormalities of the hemostatic system can contribute to bleeding during liver surgery. Hemostatic function is determined by the interaction of the vascular wall, platelets, coagulation factors, and fibrinolytic function. All these components of the hemostatic system may be abnormal in patients who have a compromised liver function, and this may contribute to excessive bleeding during liver surgery.[8,9] However, despite the multiple laboratory abnormalities in the hemostatic system, patients who have cirrhosis can nowadays undergo major surgical procedures such as liver transplantation or partial liver resection without transfusion of blood products.[9] Although part of this can be explained by important advances in surgical methods and techniques, it may also imply that the detected abnormalities in laboratory tests of the hemostatic system are (not always) clinically relevant. Indeed, several investigators have shown that preoperative conventional coagulation assays are a poor predictor of blood loss during liver transplantation.[10,11] In addition, the correction of a prolonged prothrombin time with

Department of Surgery, Section of Hepatobiliary Surgery and Liver Transplantation, University Medical Center Groningen, University of Groningen, P.O. Box 30.001, 9700 RB Groningen, The Netherlands
* Corresponding author.
E-mail address: r.j.porte@chir.umcg.nl (R.J. Porte).

Clin Liver Dis 13 (2009) 145–154
doi:10.1016/j.cld.2008.09.012
1089-3261/08/$ – see front matter © 2009 Elsevier Inc. All rights reserved.

liver.theclinics.com

recombinant factor VIIa has not been shown to lead to a reduction in blood loss or transfusion requirements in patients undergoing major liver surgery.[12,13]

The main progress in reducing perioperative blood loss has been made through improved surgical and anesthetic techniques and through better understanding of hemostatic disorders in patients who have liver disease.[7,14] The purpose of this article is to provide a clinically oriented guide to the prevention and treatment of bleeding in liver surgery. The authors discuss the developments in surgical, anesthesiologic, and pharmacologic strategies that have contributed to a reduction of blood loss during liver surgery in cirrhotic and noncirrhotic patients. The clinical relevance of different types of strategies may vary, depending on the stage of the operation. For example, topical hemostatic agents have a role in reducing blood loss from the hepatic resection surface after partial liver resection, whereas surgical techniques play a more important role during transsection of the liver parenchyma (**Fig. 1**).

SURGICAL STRATEGIES TO REDUCE BLOOD LOSS

Refinements in surgical techniques and better understanding of the liver anatomy have provided important contributions to the reduction of blood loss during liver surgery. In recent years, several new techniques have been developed to perform more complex surgical interventions in patients who have a pre-existing bleeding risk, such as patients who have liver cirrhosis (**Box 1**). In addition, improvements in the preoperative imaging and evaluation of the liver function reserve have contributed to a better selection of patients and a lower overall postoperative morbidity and mortality.[15,16]

Blood loss during a partial liver resection may vary during the three stages of the procedure (see **Fig. 1**). The first stage, in which the efferent and afferent vessels of the part of the liver that needs to be resected are identified, is characterized by minor

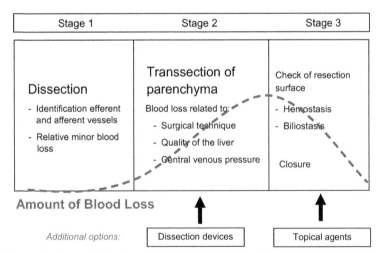

Fig. 1. The mechanisms of bleeding and the relative amount of blood loss (*dotted line*) during the three surgical stages of partial liver resections. In general, most bleeding can be encountered during transsection of the liver parenchyma. In this stage of the operation, blood loss is mainly caused by bleeding from the resection surface of the liver. Volume contraction and a low intravascular filling status (ie, low central venous pressure) are generally more effective in reducing blood loss in this stage than massive transfusion of blood products such as fresh-frozen plasma.

Box 1
Surgical and anesthesiologic methods used to reduce blood loss in liver surgery

Surgical

Vascular clamping techniques

    Inflow occlusion

        Continuous Pringle maneuver

        Continuous Pringle maneuver after ischemic preconditioning

        Intermittent Pringle maneuver

    Total vascular occlusion

Dissection devices for transsection of liver parenchyma

    Classic methods

        Scalpel

        "Finger-fracture" method

        Clamp crushing

    Ultrasonic dissection

    Hydro-jet dissection

    Electro coagulation (Argon coagulation)

    Radiofrequency ablation-based devices

Topic hemostatic agents

Anesthesiologic

Maintaining low central venous pressure by using

    Volume contraction

    Phlebotomy

    Vasodilatation

    If needed, forced diuresis

Blood products

Use of pharmacologic agents

    Antifibrinolytics

    Recombinant factor VIIa

---

blood loss. An exception may be patients who have intra-abdominal adhesions caused by previous abdominal surgery and patients who have significant portal hypertension, who generally have a higher bleeding tendency. In general, the amount of surgical blood loss is the highest in the second stage of liver resection, when transsection of the parenchyma is performed. In this stage, the quality of the liver tissue, the dissection method used, and the central venous pressure (CVP) may influence the extent of blood loss. Selective vascular occlusion techniques have an important role in controlling blood loss in this stage of the operation, as was recently discussed elsewhere.[17–20] Van der Belt and colleagues[20] studied the application of vascular occlusion methods by sending a questionnaire to 621 surgeons in Europe. Although the overall response rate was low (50%), this study provided good insight into current practice. Most of the responding surgeons indicated that clamping of the liver vasculature is used selectively when excessive blood loss occurs during hepatic resection. Complete inflow occlusion (ie, the Pringle maneuver) is the most frequently applied method in this situation. Similar results have been reported by Nakajima and colleagues,[21] based on a survey of 231 hospitals in Japan. A disadvantage of using vascular inflow occlusion is the resulting ischemic injury of the liver. Intermittent clamping or ischemic preconditioning may decrease the amount of ischemic injury, especially in cirrhotic livers.[21,22] However, intermittent clamping is also associated with more bleeding than continuous clamping.[22] Nevertheless, it is the most frequently applied method of vascular occlusion in Europe.[20]

In addition to vascular inflow occlusion techniques, several new methods and devices for transsection of the liver parenchyma have been developed (see **Box 1**). The Cavitron Ultrasonic Surgical Aspirator (CUSA) is the most frequently used device, followed by precoagulation devices.[20,21] Although most of these devices may contribute to a reduction of blood loss during the transsection phase, some of them perform slowly and some groups have reported disappointing results.[22,23] In a prospective randomized clinical trial, Lesurtel and colleagues[24] compared four techniques of liver transsection in 100 noncirrhotic patients undergoing major liver resections. The conventional clamp-crashing technique was compared with CUSA, Hydro-jet, and a dissecting sealer.[25] In this study, the clamp-crashing technique was associated with significantly lower blood loss, shorter resection time, and lower costs, compared with the other three techniques. So, all in all, the beneficial effects of these new devices are not entirely clear and more prospective studies will be needed to assess the role of these devices in liver surgery. In the absence of a strong advantage of any of these transsection devices, personal preference and local availability are the main factors that determine the use of a given device in a center.

ANESTHESIOLOGIC STRATEGIES TO REDUCE BLOOD LOSS

The impact of anesthesiologic care on blood loss and transfusion requirement in patients undergoing major liver surgery is mainly determined by (1) intraoperative fluid management, (2) the transfusion triggers used, and (3) the use of pharmacologic agents (the last of which will be discussed below).

Transfusion of blood products may be required in the case of active and serious bleeding, but the value of the prophylactic use of blood products, such as fresh-frozen plasma (FFP), is currently being debated.[25–27] The use of blood products, however, is highly variable and not always evidence based. For example, studies in patients undergoing liver transplantation have shown a large variability in the use of blood products among different centers and even among individual anesthesiologists within centers.[27] Although excessive bleeding may, and should, be managed by the transfusion of blood products, such as FFP, platelet concentrates, and packed red blood cells (RBC),[28] it is also becoming clear that no consensus currently exists on transfusion practice in liver surgery. Prospective, multicenter studies with predetermined hemostasis assessment and transfusion guidelines are needed and would improve our understanding of the correction and prevention of massive bleeding during liver surgery, with likely improvements in patient outcomes.[29]

In addition to monitoring and correcting blood loss and associated metabolic abnormalities, anesthesiologists play a key role in reducing blood loss during liver surgery by maintaining a low CVP. Performance of surgical practice under low CVP is one of the strategies that have been studied intensively in liver surgery.[30–33] Although already suggested by Bismuth and colleagues,[33] Jones and colleagues[32] were the first to show that blood loss during liver resection is almost linearly related to the

CVP. Low CVP (<5 mm Hg) can be achieved by applying volume contraction, by using vasodilating agents, or by stimulation of forced diuresis (see **Box 1**). Volume contraction has been suggested as a safe method of reducing blood loss during liver surgery. It can be achieved by a restrictive use of fluid and blood products, avoidance of fluid overload, and no routine correction of abnormal coagulation tests by infusion of FFP or other large-volume blood products.[2,4,31] Although a low CVP is associated with reduced blood loss, it also carries a higher risk for complications such as air embolism, systemic tissue hypoperfusion, and renal failure.[2,30,34,35] Schroeder and colleagues[34] studied the safety of a fluid restriction policy and low CVP in liver transplant recipients by comparing outcome variables in two centers with different policies. One center had the policy to aim for a low CVP (<5 mm Hg) by using fluid restriction, whereas the second center did not take any specific measures to lower the CVP and aimed for normal CVP policy (7–10 mm Hg). Both patient groups were similar in demographics, cause of liver disease, and surgical methods. The low CVP group received lower amounts of RBC (3.8 versus 11.6 units, $P<.01$), FFP (1.3 versus 14.7 units, $P<.001$), and platelets (0.6 versus 2.4 units, $P<.001$) compared with the normal CVP group. However, the postoperative peak serum creatinine level (3.2 versus 1.8 mg/dL, $P<.01$), the need for dialysis (6.8% versus 1.2%, $P<.05$), and 30-day mortality (6 [8.2%] versus 0, $P<.05$) were higher in patients who had low CVP. A limitation of this study is the lack of randomization and the comparison of two centers, which may have differed in many other aspects than just a CVP target. Contrary to the study by Schroeder and colleagues, Wang and colleagues[36] found no detrimental effect on maintaining a low CVP in a prospective study of 50 cirrhotic patients undergoing partial liver resection for hepatocellular carcinoma. Patients were divided into an intervention group (n = 25), in which the CVP was maintained at less than or equal to 4 mm Hg, and a control group (n = 25) with normal CVP. Intraoperative blood loss was significantly lower in the group with low CVP, compared with the control group (903 ± 180 mL versus 2329 ± 2538 mL, $P<.01$). In addition, RBC and FFP transfusion requirements were significantly lower and hospital stay was shorter in the group with low CVP, whereas no negative effect was found in postoperative hepatic and renal function.

Some groups have taken the concept of fluid contraction much further than only reducing fluid infusions, and these groups even performed phlebotomy as a strategy to minimize intraoperative blood loss in patients undergoing major liver surgery.[35,37] Hashimoto and colleagues[37] performed a randomized controlled trial in 79 healthy participants who underwent partial liver resection for living donor liver transplantation. Participants were randomly allocated to a blood withdrawal group (n = 40, collecting a volume of blood corresponding to 0.7% of the patient's body weight) or a control group (n = 39) with no blood withdrawal. Surgeons were blinded for the allocated groups. The CVP at the beginning of the parenchymal transsection was significantly lower in the group with blood withdrawal (median 5 [range 2–9] cm H_2O versus 6 [range 2–13] cm H_2O, $P = .005$) compared with controls. Blood loss during liver transsection was also significantly lower in the phlebotomized group (140 [range 40–430] mL versus 230 [range 40–660] mL, $P = .034$). However, the two showed no statistical difference in postoperative outcomes. In another prospective study, Massicotte and colleagues[35] examined the effect of maintaining a low CVP through volume contraction and by using intraoperative phlebotomy in patients undergoing liver transplantation. Outcome in these patients was compared with outcome in a historical control group without phlebotomy.[26] Intraoperative blood loss was significantly lower in the prospective group with a low CVP (903 ± 582 mL versus 1479 ± 1750 mL, $P = .001$), and no patient required dialysis in the postoperative period.

In general, evidence is increasing that blood loss during major liver surgery is strongly influenced by the filling status and CVP of the patient. Measures to reduce the filling status of the patient and to lower the CVP through volume contraction and no routine correction of laboratory coagulation test with large-volume blood products is effective and safe. Larger prospective studies will be needed to define the exact role and safety of blood withdrawal as a measure of reducing the CVP and minimizing blood loss during liver surgery.

PHARMACOLOGIC STRATEGIES TO REDUCE BLOOD LOSS

Several pharmacologic measures are available to treat or prevent bleeding complications during liver surgery. However, these agents should only be used as complementary to other methods in reducing blood loss. Three main categories can be recognized: topical hemostatic agents, antifibrinolytic drugs, and procoagulant drugs.[38]

Topical Hemostatic Agents

Topical agents may be useful to stimulate hemostasis at the resection surface of the liver after parenchymal transsection. Based on their working mechanism, topical agents can be divided into three groups: agents that mimic coagulation (ie, fibrin sealants), agents that provide a matrix for endogenous coagulation (ie, collagen, gelatin, and cellulose sponges), and combined products that work as a matrix for endogenous and exogenous coagulation factors.[38,39] Current scientific evidence suggests beneficial effects in reducing the time to hemostasis and in lowering the requirements for perioperative RBC transfusions.[39–43] Although the beneficial effects of fibrin sealants have also been confirmed in a recent Cochrane review,[44] the efficacy of fibrin sealant in liver surgery has recently been questioned.[45] In a large, randomized, controlled trial in 300 patients undergoing partial liver resection, Figueras and associates[45] found no difference in total blood loss, transfusion requirements, or postoperative morbidity between patients treated with fibrin sealants (n = 150) and a control group without fibrin sealants (n = 150).

Antifibrinolytics

Antifibrinolytics can be categorized into two groups: inhibitors of plasminogen (lysine analogs tranexamic acid and epsilon-aminocaproic acid), and inhibitors of plasmin (serine protease inhibitors aprotinin and nafamostat mesylate). In recent years, several studies and reviews have been published on the efficacy and safety of antifibrinolytics in liver surgery and transplantation.[14,38,46–49] In liver transplantation, aprotinin and tranexamic acid have been shown to result in a significant reduction in blood loss and transfusion requirements of around 30% to 40%.[50] Because of recent safety concerns, especially a higher risk for renal failure and perioperative death in patients who were given aprotinin during cardiac surgery, marketing of aprotinin has recently been suspended. However, in the liver transplant population, prospective studies have not caused any safety concerns, and no increased risk for thromboembolic events or renal failure has been noted in liver transplant patients treated with aprotinin.[50,51] Although antifibrinolytics have been studied extensively in liver transplantation, only two prospective studies have examined the efficacy in patients undergoing liver resections.[52,53] In general, improvements in surgical technique and anesthesiologic care seem to be more important in reducing blood loss in patients undergoing partial liver resections than the use of the antifibrinolytic drugs. Antifibrinolytics may be indicated in a selected group of patients who have cirrhosis and are undergoing liver resection, but further studies in this specific group of patients will be needed.[54]

Procoagulant Drugs

The efficacy and safety of the recombinant factor VIIa has been studied in several randomized clinical trials in cirrhotic and noncirrhotic patients undergoing partial liver resections or transplantation.[12,13,55–57] Although these studies did not cause major safety concerns,[38,58,59] they also failed to demonstrate a significant difference in blood loss or transfusion requirements between patients who received recombinant factor VIIa or placebo. In all of these studies, recombinant factor VIIa was used as a prophylactic drug, which may not be the most efficient use for this drug. Probably, this drug should be seen more as a drug that can be used a "rescue therapy" to control bleeding in situations of major bleeding where other therapies have failed. More research in this area is needed.

SUMMARY

In general, perioperative blood loss and blood transfusions have a negative impact on postoperative outcome after liver surgery. Surgical technique and experience are key factors determining the amount of blood loss in liver surgery. Inflow occlusion (the Pringle maneuver) and the use of low CVP are simple and effective measures of reducing blood loss during parenchyma transsection. No superiority of one dissection device has been shown above the others, and their use depends mainly on the quality of the liver parenchyma and personal preference and experience. The emerging evidence indicates that abnormal coagulation tests do not predict bleeding in cirrhotic patients. Preprocedural correction of coagulation tests with blood products has not been shown to reduce intraoperative bleeding and it even seems counterproductive because it results mainly in an increase of the intravascular filling status of the patient, which may, in fact, enhance the bleeding risk. Factors such as portal hypertension and the hyperdynamic circulation in patients who have cirrhosis may play a more important role in the bleeding tendency of these patients. Therefore, volume contraction, rather than prophylactic transfusion blood products (ie, FFP), seems justified in patients undergoing major liver surgery. An increasing number of studies suggest that volume contraction in these patients is safe and effective in reducing perioperative blood loss and transfusion requirements. Although antifibrinolytic drugs proved to be effective in reducing blood loss during liver transplantation, topical or systemic hemostatic drugs are of limited value in reducing blood loss in patients undergoing partial liver resections.

REFERENCES

1. Hendriks HG, van der MJ, De Wolf JT, et al. Intraoperative blood transfusion requirement is the main determinant of early surgical re-intervention after orthotopic liver transplantation. Transpl Int 2005;17:673–9.
2. Cacciarelli TV, Keeffe EB, Moore DH, et al. Effect of intraoperative blood transfusion on patient outcome in hepatic transplantation. Arch Surg 1999;134:25–9.
3. Stainsby D, Williamson L, Jones H, et al. 6 Years of shot reporting–its influence on UK blood safety. Transfus Apheresis Sci 2004;31:123–31.
4. de Boer MT, Molenaar IQ, Hendriks HG, et al. Minimizing blood loss in liver transplantation: progress through research and evolution of techniques. Dig Surg 2005;22:265–75.

5. Porte RJ, Hendriks HG, Slooff MJ. Blood conservation in liver transplantation: the role of aprotinin. J Cardiothorac Vasc Anesth 2004;18:31S–7S.
6. Ramos E, Dalmau A, Sabate A, et al. Intraoperative red blood cell transfusion in liver transplantation: influence on patient outcome, prediction of requirements, and measures to reduce them. Liver Transpl 2003;9:1320–7.
7. Marietta M, Facchini L, Pedrazzi P, et al. Pathophysiology of bleeding in surgery. Transplant Proc 2006;38(3):812–4. Ref Type: Hearing.
8. Porte RJ, Knot EA, Bontempo FA. Hemostasis in liver transplantation. Gastroenterology 1989;97:488–501.
9. Lisman T, Leebeek FW. Hemostatic alterations in liver disease: a review on pathophysiology, clinical consequences, and treatment. Dig Surg 2007;24:250–8.
10. Findlay JY, Rettke SR. Poor prediction of blood transfusion requirements in adult liver transplantations from preoperative variables. J Clin Anesth 2000;12:319–23.
11. Steib A, Freys G, Lehmann C, et al. Intraoperative blood losses and transfusion requirements during adult liver transplantation remain difficult to predict. Can J Anaesth 2001;48:1075–9.
12. Lodge JP, Jonas S, Oussoultzoglou E, et al. Recombinant coagulation factor VIIa in major liver resection: a randomized, placebo-controlled, double-blind clinical trial. Anesthesiology 2005;102:269–75.
13. Planinsic RM, van der MJ, Testa G, et al. Safety and efficacy of a single bolus administration of recombinant factor VIIa in liver transplantation due to chronic liver disease. Liver Transpl 2005;11:895–900.
14. Groenland TH, Porte RJ. Antifibrinolytics in liver transplantation. Int Anesthesiol Clin 2006;44:83–97.
15. Friedman LS. The risk of surgery in patients with liver disease. Hepatology 1999;29:1617–23.
16. Suman A, Carey WD. Assessing the risk of surgery in patients with liver disease. Cleve Clin J Med 2006;73:398–404.
17. van Gulik TM, de GW, Dinant S, et al. Vascular occlusion techniques during liver resection. Dig Surg 2007;24:274–81.
18. Smyrniotis V, Farantos C, Kostopanagiotou G, et al. Vascular control during hepatectomy: review of methods and results. World J Surg 2005;29:1384–96.
19. Dixon E, Vollmer CM Jr, Bathe OF, et al. Vascular occlusion to decrease blood loss during hepatic resection. Am J Surg 2005;190:75–86.
20. van der Bilt JD, Livestro DP, Borren A, et al. European survey on the application of vascular clamping in liver surgery. Dig Surg 2007;24:423–35.
21. Nakajima Y, Shimamura T, Kamiyama T, et al. Control of intraoperative bleeding during liver resection: analysis of a questionnaire sent to 231 Japanese hospitals. Surg Today 2002;32:48–52.
22. Selzner N, Rudiger H, Graf R, et al. Protective strategies against ischemic injury of the liver. Gastroenterology 2003;125:917–36.
23. Takayama T, Makuuchi M, Kubota K, et al. Randomized comparison of ultrasonic vs clamp transection of the liver. Arch Surg 2001;136:922–8.
24. Lesurtel M, Selzner M, Petrowsky H, et al. How should transection of the liver be performed?: a prospective randomized study in 100 consecutive patients: comparing four different transection strategies. Ann Surg 2005;242:814–22 [discussion].
25. Lisman T, Caldwell SH, Porte RJ, et al. Consequences of abnormal hemostasis tests for clinical practice. J Thromb Haemost 2006;4:2062–3.

26. Massicotte L, Sassine MP, Lenis S, et al. Transfusion predictors in liver transplant. Anesth Analg 2004;98:1245–51, table.
27. Ozier Y, Pessione F, Samain E, et al. Institutional variability in transfusion practice for liver transplantation. Anesth Analg 2003;97:671–9.
28. Kang Y, Audu P. Coagulation and liver transplantation. Int Anesthesiol Clin 2006; 44:17–36.
29. Lopez-Plaza I. Transfusion guidelines and liver transplantation: time for consensus. Liver Transpl 2007;13:1630–2.
30. Melendez JA, Arslan V, Fischer ME, et al. Perioperative outcomes of major hepatic resections under low central venous pressure anesthesia: blood loss, blood transfusion, and the risk of postoperative renal dysfunction. J Am Coll Surg 1998;187:620–5.
31. Smyrniotis V, Kostopanagiotou G, Theodoraki K, et al. The role of central venous pressure and type of vascular control in blood loss during major liver resections. Am J Surg 2004;187:398–402.
32. Jones RM, Moulton CE, Hardy KJ. Central venous pressure and its effect on blood loss during liver resection. Br J Surg 1998;85:1058–60.
33. Bismuth H, Castaing D, Garden OJ. Major hepatic resection under total vascular exclusion. Ann Surg 1989;210:13–9.
34. Schroeder RA, Collins BH, Tuttle-Newhall E, et al. Intraoperative fluid management during orthotopic liver transplantation. J Cardiothorac Vasc Anesth 2004; 18:438–41.
35. Massicotte L, Lenis S, Thibeault L, et al. Effect of low central venous pressure and phlebotomy on blood product transfusion requirements during liver transplantations. Liver Transpl 2006;12:117–23.
36. Wang WD, Liang LJ, Huang XQ, et al. Low central venous pressure reduces blood loss in hepatectomy. World J Gastroenterol 2006;12:935–9.
37. Hashimoto T, Kokudo N, Orii R, et al. Intraoperative blood salvage during liver resection: a randomized controlled trial. Ann Surg 2007;245:686–91.
38. Porte RJ, Leebeek FW. Pharmacological strategies to decrease transfusion requirements in patients undergoing surgery. Drugs 2002;62:2193–211.
39. Berrevoet F, de HB. Use of topical hemostatic agents during liver resection. Dig Surg 2007;24:288–93.
40. Heaton N. Advances and methods in liver surgery: haemostasis. Eur J Gastroenterol Hepatol 2005;17(Suppl 1):S3–12.
41. Chapman WC, Clavien PA, Fung J, et al. Effective control of hepatic bleeding with a novel collagen-based composite combined with autologous plasma: results of a randomized controlled trial. Arch Surg 2000;135: 1200–4.
42. Schwartz M, Madariaga J, Hirose R, et al. Comparison of a new fibrin sealant with standard topical hemostatic agents. Arch Surg 2004;139: 1148–54.
43. Jackson MR. Fibrin sealants in surgical practice: an overview. Am J Surg 2001; 182:1S–7S.
44. Carless PA, Henry DA, Anthony DM. Fibrin sealant use for minimising peri-operative allogeneic blood transfusion. Cochrane Database Syst Rev 2003;1: CD004171.
45. Figueras J, Llado L, Miro M, et al. Application of fibrin glue sealant after hepatectomy does not seem justified: results of a randomized study in 300 patients. Ann Surg 2007;245:536–42.

46. Xia VW, Steadman RH. Antifibrinolytics in orthotopic liver transplantation: current status and controversies. Liver Transpl 2005;11:10–8.

47. Ozier Y, Schlumberger S. Pharmacological approaches to reducing blood loss and transfusions in the surgical patient. Can J Anaesth 2006;53:S21–9.

48. Henry DA, Carless PA, Moxey AJ, et al. Anti-fibrinolytic use for minimising perioperative allogeneic blood transfusion. Cochrane Database Syst Rev 2007;4: CD001886.

49. Dalmau A, Sabate A, Acosta F, et al. Tranexamic acid reduces red cell transfusion better than epsilon-aminocaproic acid or placebo in liver transplantation. Anesth Analg 2000;91:29–34.

50. Molenaar IQ, Warnaar N, Groen H, et al. Efficacy and safety of antifibrinolytic drugs in liver transplantation: a systematic review and meta-analysis. Am J Transplant 2007;7:185–94.

51. Warnaar N, Mallett SV, de Boer MT, et al. The impact of aprotinin on renal function after liver transplantation: an analysis of 1,043 patients. Am J Transplant 2007;7: 2378–87.

52. Lentschener C, Benhamou D, Mercier FJ, et al. Aprotinin reduces blood loss in patients undergoing elective liver resection. Anesth Analg 1997;84:875–81.

53. Wu CC, Ho WM, Cheng SB, et al. Perioperative parenteral tranexamic acid in liver tumor resection: a prospective randomized trial toward a "blood transfusion"-free hepatectomy. Ann Surg 2006;243:173–80.

54. Pereboom IT, de Boer MT, Porte RJ, et al. Aprotinin and nafamostat mesilate in liver surgery: effect on blood loss. Dig Surg 2007;24:282–7.

55. Lodge JP, Jonas S, Jones RM, et al. Efficacy and safety of repeated perioperative doses of recombinant factor VIIa in liver transplantation. Liver Transpl 2005;11: 973–9.

56. Hendriks HG, Meijer K, de Wolf JT, et al. Reduced transfusion requirements by recombinant factor VIIa in orthotopic liver transplantation: a pilot study. Transplantation 2001;71:402–5.

57. Meijer K, Hendriks HG, de Wolf JT, et al. Recombinant factor VIIa in orthotopic liver transplantation: influence on parameters of coagulation and fibrinolysis. Blood Coagul Fibrinolysis 2003;14:169–74.

58. Vincent JL, Rossaint R, Riou B, et al. Recommendations on the use of recombinant activated factor VII as an adjunctive treatment for massive bleeding–a European perspective. Crit Care 2006;10(4):R120.

59. Levy JH, Fingerhut A, Brott T, et al. Recombinant factor VIIa in patients with coagulopathy secondary to anticoagulant therapy, cirrhosis, or severe traumatic injury: review of safety profile. Transfusion 2006;46:919–33.

Coagulation Disorders and Bleeding in Liver Disease: Future Directions

Stephen H. Caldwell, MD[a],*, Arun J. Sanyal, MD[b]

KEYWORDS

- Coagulation • Bleeding • Cirrhosis • Liver disease
- Hyperfibrinolysis • Dysfibrinogen • Heparinoids

From the foregoing articles, it is evident that several long-held tenets regarding the pathophysiology and assessment of coagulopathy in liver disease are undergoing scrutiny and revision. Among the most important concepts to emerge over the past few years is that the typical cirrhotic patient has multiple and frequently opposing factors that influence hemostasis and clot formation and, perhaps most importantly, that the conventional international normalized ratio (INR) is a limited measure of this disturbance, especially in terms of predicting adequate, excessive, or inadequate clot formation. Coupled with the limitations and risks associated with blood product infusion, this situation calls into question many common clinical practices and increases the need for clinical and laboratory-based investigation.

BLEEDING RISK ASSESSMENT

Bleeding risk assessment affects many day-to-day aspects of the clinical practice of hepatology, from the mundane rescheduling of a procedure because of a prolonged INR to life-threatening anasarca or transfusion-associated lung injury, with the excessive and often counterproductive administration of plasma. The use of plasma to correct INR preprocedure to some arbitrary number, however, completely misses the pathways measured by this test and the pathophysiology leading to its prolongation. One example is its use in a patient in liver failure from initially unrecognized Budd-Chiari syndrome whose INR was prolonged to 9 seconds but whose research thromboelastogram clearly identified a hypercoagulable state.

[a] GI/Hepatology Division, Digestive Health Center of Excellence, University of Virginia Medical Center, Box 800708, Charlottesville, VA 22908 0708, USA
[b] Division of GI/Hepatology and Nutrition, Department of Internal Medicine, VCU School of Medicine, MCV Box 980341, Richmond, VA 23298 0341, USA
* Corresponding author.
E-mail address: shc5c@virginia.edu (S.H. Caldwell).

Clin Liver Dis 13 (2009) 155–157
doi:10.1016/j.cld.2008.09.011
1089-3261/08/$ – see front matter © 2009 Elsevier Inc. All rights reserved.

liver.theclinics.com

Clearly, patients who have liver failure, whether acute or acute-on-chronic failure, may have serious bleeding problems. A pressing need exists to develop, validate, and disseminate a global measure of coagulation that is clinically meaningful. Some candidate tests that are under evaluation include thromboelastography, endogenous thrombin generation, and platelet function. In other words, translational research is essential to apply the recent laboratory advances, to define more precisely where a given patient is in terms of coagulation and hemostasis and thus how to apply the most appropriate management strategy. Indeed, inappropriate reliance on the INR and failure to risk stratify bleeding risk effectively in cirrhosis may explain, in part, the variable results seen in many of the recombinant factor VIIa trials over the past 10 years (see the article by Shah and colleagues elsewhere in this issue).

BLOOD PRODUCT AND PROCOAGULANT USE IN CIRRHOSIS

It is increasingly recognized that changes in conventional patterns of blood product use in clinical practice are warranted. However, to define such an undertaking better, it is helpful to understand how these products are being used in current practice. To this end, efforts are underway to measure total blood product use in patients who have liver disease at multiple centers around the world, to assess common practices and to determine variation in practice and assess indications and outcomes of their use. It is hoped that such a "snapshot" of current practice will provide some guidance in the development of clinical investigation to "translate" recent laboratory advances into improved clinical care.

IMPLEMENTATION OF THE INTERNATIONAL NORMALIZED RATIO$_{LIVER}$?

Two studies from centers in Italy and France (see article by Tripodi and colleagues in this issue) have independently demonstrated the usefulness of a new version of the INR that is free of the coumadin-based reference range.[1,2] It takes into account many of the unique aspects of the coagulopathy of liver disease and it results in remarkable reproducibility. Thus, the prospect seems feasible of eradicating the significant interlaboratory variation in INR and, hence, in the Model for End-Stage Liver Disease (MELD) score that Trotter and colleagues have demonstrated in the United States (see article by Arjal and Trotter in this issue) and which has been more recently demonstrated in Europe by Lisman and colleagues.[3,4] However, proponents of the MELD score, although acknowledging the potential usefulness of the INR$_{liver}$, note the excellent performance of the MELD score using the conventional INR and the difficulty in implementing a new standard. Nonetheless, the prospect of significant variation of the MELD (up to 20%) using the conventional INR, and the implications of this situation for organ allocation, warrant efforts to develop the INR$_{liver}$ as the new standard by which MELD is measured, which clearly presents a challenge in implementing a broad change in laboratory practice. However, the growing impact on health care of chronic liver disease due to viral hepatitis, nonalcoholic steatohepatitis, and alcohol-related liver disease support the need to address this problem effectively.

PROGRESSION OF CIRRHOSIS DUE TO PARENCHYMAL EXTINCTION

Cirrhosis, which is commonly tagged with the adjective "end-stage," is often a stable condition, potentially for many years. Several developments can underlie deterioration of stable cirrhosis to the state commonly referred to as "decompensated cirrhosis." Liver atrophy is often an associated finding in this state, which usually does represent an "end-stage" condition. Wanless and colleagues were the first to demonstrate the role of prothrombotic conditions in causing diffuse atrophy through a process they called "parenchymal extinction" (see the articles by Anstee and colleagues and North-up in this issue).[5] The mechanisms involved appear to be more complex than simple stasis and clot formation, although these may certainly contribute. Rather, the process may also involve thrombin-related signaling pathways and possibly platelet activation. Recognition of this process as a common means by which cirrhosis progresses raises the prospect of some form of anticoagulation as a means of preventing organ atrophy. Further studies of this provocative strategy are clearly warranted.

SUMMARY

Much has changed since the seminal paper of Boks and colleagues, which demon-strated the wide spectrum of abnormalities in the coagulation system in patients who have acute and chronic liver disease and the possible role of hyperfibrinolysis in bleeding in many of these patients.[6] With a growing number of therapeutic options and increasing recognition of the inherent limitations of conventional laboratory mea-sures of coagulation in the patient who has liver disease, it is now incumbent on us to explore how best to apply (or withhold) specific agents in specific situations. This ex-ploration will clearly require well-focused translational research to understand and bring into sharp focus the various problems present, from dysfibrinogen to endoge-nous heparinoids, to uremia, to hypercoagulable conditions. The challenge lies ahead.

REFERENCES

1. Tripodi A. How to implement the modified international normalized ratio for cirrho-sis (INR(liver)) for model for end-stage liver disease calculation. Hepatology 2008; 47:1423–4.
2. Bellest L, Eschwege V, Poupon R, et al. A modified international normalized ratio as an effective way of prothrombin time standardization in hepatology. Hepatology 2007;46:528–34.
3. Trotter JF, Olson J, Lefkowitz J, et al. Changes in international normalized ratio (INR) and Model for End-Stage Liver Disease (MELD) based on selection of clin-ical laboratory. Am J Transpl 2007;7:1624–8.
4. Lisman T, van Leeuwen Y, Adelmeijer J, et al. Interlaboratory variability in assess-ment of the model of end-stage liver disease score. Liver International 2008;28: 1344–51.
5. Wanless IR, Wong F, Blendis LM, et al. Hepatic and portal vein thrombosis in cirrhosis: possible role in development of parenchymal extinction and portal hypertension. Hepatology 1995;21:1238–47.
6. Boks AL, Brommer EJ, Schalm SW, et al. Hemostasis and fibrinolysis in severe liver failure and their relation to hemorrhage. Hepatology 1986;6:79–86.

Index

Note: Page numbers of article titles are in **boldface** type.

A

Activated partial thromboplastin time, in coagulation testing in liver disease, 56–57
Acute liver failure
    coagulopathy of, **95–107**
        clinical presentation of, 97–98
            bleeding during and after OLT, 98
            iatrogenic bleeding, 98
            spontaneous bleeding, 97
        described, 95
        frequency of, 95–96
        laboratory evaluation of, 98–100
        management of, 100–103
        pathophysiology of, 96–97
    described, 95
    severity of, 95–96
Anemia, in cirrhosis, 35
Anesthesia/anesthetics, in blood loss management in liver surgery, 148–150
Antifibrinolytic(s)
    in blood loss management in liver surgery, 150–151
    in ESLD management, 89–91

B

Bleeding
    during and after OLT, in coagulopathy of acute renal failure, 98
    hyperfibrinolysis and, 23
    iatrogenic, in coagulopathy of acute renal failure, 98
    in liver disease
        future directions in, **155–157**
        risk assessment for, 155–156
    in liver surgery, **145–154**
        described, 145–146
        management of, strategies to reduce blood loss in
            anesthesiologic, 148–150
            pharmacologic, 150–151
            surgical, 146–148
    risk factors associated with, 14–15
    spontaneous, in coagulopathy of acute renal failure, 97
Bleeding diathesis, in cirrhosis, 76–78
Bleeding time, platelet aggregation and, 14–15

Clin Liver Dis 13 (2009) 159–166
doi:10.1016/S1089-3261(08)00128-1

Printed and bound by CPI Group (UK) Ltd, Croydon, CR0 4YY

03/10/2024

01040444-0010

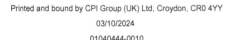